Risk and citizenship

Key issues in welfare

Edited by
Rosalind Edwards and
Judith Glover

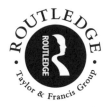

London and New York

First published 2001
by Routledge
11 New Fetter Lane, London EC4P 4EE

Simultaneously published in the USA and Canada
by Routledge
29 West 35th Street, New York, NY 10001

Routledge is an imprint of the Taylor & Francis Group

Typeset in Times by Keystroke, Jacaranda Lodge, Wolverhampton
Printed and bound in Great Britain by Biddles Ltd, Guildford and
King's Lynn

British Library Cataloguing in Publication Data
A catalogue record for this book is available from the British Library

Library of Congress Cataloging in Publication Data
A catalog record for this book has been requested

ISBN 0–415–24158–8 (hbk)
ISBN 0–415–24159–6 (pbk)

Risk and citizenship

Contemporary welfare provision poses serious challenges for social policy. Large
vork and relate

of citizenship
cations for the
t provides:

re
and community

ysts addresses
: the nature of
egalitarianism;
s of citizenship;
nd citizenship
y-maker.

esearch Centre,
Sociology and

Contents

Figures and tables

Figures

Tables

Notes on contributors

David Abbott is a researcher at the Norah Fry Research Centre, University of Bristol where he is currently working on projects relating to the lives of disabled children. The fieldwork described in his chapter with Deborah Quilgars was carried out when he worked at the Centre for Research in Social Policy at Loughborough University.

Ann Davis is Professor of Social Work in the Department of Social Policy and Social Work, the University of Birmingham. She has particular interests in issues of user experiences of social work, community care, poverty and social exclusion. She has researched and written on these subjects.

Rosalind Edwards is Professor in Social Policy at South Bank University. She has carried out research on a variety of family policy issues, including mothers and education; lone and partnered mothers, employment and child care; step-families; and children's understandings of parental involvement in education. Her recent publications include: *Feminist Dilemmas in Qualitative Research: Public Knowledge and Private Lives* (co-edited with J. Ribbens, Sage, 1998) and *Lone Mothers, Paid Work and Gendered Moral Rationalities* (with S. Duncan, Macmillan, 1999). She co-edits (with J. Brannen) *The International Journal of Social Research Methodology: Theory and Practice*.

Kathryn Ellis is Senior Lecturer in Social Policy at the University of Luton. Her research interests include community care, disability policy and politics, social policy and the body, women and social welfare. Her most recent book is *Social Policy and the Body: Transitions in Corporeal Discourse* (ed. with H. Dean, Macmillan, 1999).

Zsuzsa Ferge is an economist, having worked in the field of social statistics, sociology and social policy, and became Professor of Sociology at Eotvos University in Budapest in 1988. She founded the first department of social policy in Hungary in 1989 and is still teaching there. Her main fields of interest in research and teaching are social structure, social inequalities, poverty, and the social impact of transition. She has been visiting professor at universities in France, the UK and USA. She is a member of the European Academy and of the Hungarian Academy of Sciences, and has an honorary degree from Edinburgh University. She has published around 15 books and over 200 papers.

Judith Glover is Reader in Social Policy at University of Surrey Roehampton. Her research interests focus on women's employment, studied in both the UK and cross-nationally. She has a particular substantive interest in women in scientific education and employment, and a methodological interest in the secondary analysis of large data sets. She has published on these interests in journals such as *Work, Employment and Society, Gender, Work and Organisations* and *Sociétés Contemporaines*. She is the author of *Women and Scientific Employment* (Macmillan, 1999).

Barbara Jones is Senior Research Fellow and member of the Innovation Studies and Evaluation research group (ISERg) in the Faculty of Social Sciences, Manchester Metropolitan University. Her current research interests include the political economy of technological change and innovation: economics of networks including sectoral and labour market studies and the relationship between work, education and training in new technology areas.

Ruth Lister is Professor of Social Policy in the Department of Social Sciences, Loughborough University. She is a former Director of the Child Poverty Action Group and has published widely around poverty, income maintenance and citizenship. Her latest book is *Citizenship: Feminist Perspectives* (Macmillan, 1997).

John Macnicol is Professor of Social Policy at Royal Holloway, University of London. His current research interests are the history of the 'underclass' idea, and old age, ageing and age discrimination. Recent publications include *The Politics of Retirement in Britain, 1878–1948* (Cambridge University Press, 1998) and (editor) *Paying for the Old: Old Age and Social Welfare Provision* (Thoemmes Press, 8 vols., 2000).

Bob Miller is Senior Research Fellow and member of the Innovation Studies and Evaluation Research Group (ISERg) in the Faculty of Social Sciences, Manchester Metropolitan University. His current research interests include the development of new social indicators for the information society and the effects of technological innovation on the value and survival of skills, and in the generation of new kinds of tacit knowledge in information use and knowledge generation.

Jan Pahl is Professor of Social Policy in the School of Social Policy, Sociology and Social Research at the University of Kent at Canterbury. She has carried out research on the control and allocation of money within the family, on domestic violence and on health and social care. Her publications include: *Private Violence and Public Policy* (Routledge, 1985), *Money and Marriage* (Macmillan, 1989) and *Invisible Money: Family Finances in the Electronic Economy* (Policy Press, 1999).

Deborah Quilgars is a Research Fellow in the Centre for Housing Policy at the University of York. Since joining the Centre in 1990, her research has focused on three main areas of interest: homelessness, housing and community care, and housing and risk. Along with Roger Burrows and Nicholas Pleace, Deborah co-edited *Homelessness and Social Policy* (Routledge, 1997).

David Smith is completing his Ph.D. on 'Social Exclusion and Labour Market Restructuring' at the Department of Social and Political Science, Royal Holloway, University of London.

Paul Spicker is Senior Lecturer in Social Policy at the University of Dundee. He has worked as a consultant on social policy issues, and his research has included studies related to benefit delivery systems, the care of old people, psychiatric patients, housing management and anti-poverty strategies. He has written extensively on issues relating to social policy: recent books include *Social Policy in a Changing Society* (with M. Mullard, Routledge, 1998), *The International Glossary of Poverty* (co-edited with D. Gordon, Zed Books, 1999) and *The Welfare State: A General Theory* (Sage, 2000).

Peter Taylor-Gooby is Professor of Social Policy at the University of Kent. He directed the ESRC's Economic Beliefs and Behaviour research programme. His current research is on theories of the welfare state, social welfare in the European Union and attitudes to welfare. Recent publications include: *Welfare States under Pressure* (edited, Sage, 2001), *Risk, Trust and Welfare* (edited, Macmillan, 2000), *European Welfare Futures* (with V. George and G. Bonoli, Policy Press, 2000), *Choice and Public Policy: The Limits to Welfare Markets* (edited, Macmillan, 1998), and *European Welfare Policy: Squaring the Welfare Circle* (edited with V. George, Macmillan, 1996).

Jeffrey Weeks is Professor of Sociology and Dean of Humanities and Social Science at South Bank University London. He is the author of numerous articles and 15 books, specializing on the history and social organization of sexuality. Among his publications are: *Coming Out: Homosexual Politics in Britain from the Nineteenth Century to the Present* (Quartet, 1977/1990); *Sex, Politics and Society* (Longman, 1981/1989); *Sexuality and its Discontents* (Routledge, 1985); *Sexuality* (Routledge, 1986); *Against Nature* (Rivers Oram Press, 1991); *Invented Moralities* (Polity Press, 1995); *Sexual Cultures* (ed. with Janet Holland, Macmillan, 1996); *Making Sexual History* (Polity Press, 2000); *Same Sex Intimacies: Families of Choice and Other Life Experiments* (with Brian Heaphy and Catherine Donovan, Routledge, 2001).

Chapter 1

Risk, citizenship and welfare: introduction

Rosalind Edwards and Judith Glover[1]

Introduction

Contemporary welfare provision poses serious challenges for social policy. Large and rapid changes are said to be taking place in the way we live, work and relate to each other. Long-term shifts in society have led to increasingly wider discussion of its character, with some social theorists characterizing it as 'risk society' (notably Beck 1992). Risk society is said to be marked by a pervasive and inescapable sense of concern about what is arising from past and current actions, and uncertainty about what will be encountered in the future. These shifts have resulted in debates about the nature of risk, whether and what kinds of social welfare policy interventions might reduce or modify the impact of risky events, insecurity and exclusion in such a society, and the implications for different forms of 'welfare citizenship'.

There is an impetus and a need to take stock and appraise where we are at present, reviewing these shifts in society and the thrust and impact of the social welfare policies that attempt to deal with them. For example, in the face of rapid economic, political and cultural change, is a risk-pooling approach to welfare still possible or viable? Is cultural change leading to new sorts of risks and different forms of welfare citizenship? If welfare solutions are increasingly left up to the individual, where does this leave citizens who cannot or will not self-manage welfare risks?

Several commentators have called for, or see the politics of risk society as characterized by, an active citizenship participation in democratic dialogue, so that decisions affecting citizens' welfare and the provisions made are taken in the context of informed debate (Beck 1996; Franklin 1998; Giddens 1994). This edited collection, based on papers given at the Social Policy Assocation's annual conference 'Social Insecurity and Social Policy', held at the University of Surrey Roehampton, UK, in 1999, aims to make a contribution to that informed debate. Theoretically and empirically, it addresses a range of social issues that express and reveal risk and have implications for welfare citizenship. In explicitly seeking to bring discussions of risk and citizenship together in this way, the collection throws new light on these issues and has a broader approach than texts and collections that focus on one or the other.[2]

In this introduction to the collection we aim to provide a brief review of the main features of contemporary discussions of risk and citizenship in relation to welfare, in order to provide a contextual backdrop to the more detailed discussions of particular topics presented by our contributing authors. It is not our intention to produce a comprehensive account of all the intricacies of debates, arguments and counter-arguments, concerning risk and citizenship as distinct topics (and allied concepts such as individualization and social exclusion). Rather, we are drawing attention to the contours of each of these issues as they interrelate with implications for welfare provision. This is one of the reasons why we use the (slightly contrived) term 'welfare citizenship'. We are signalling our concern with the implications and impact of risk society for and on relations between individuals and the state, and between (individual and communal) citizens with respect to welfare provisions. Having said this however, we recognize that 'welfare citizenship' fundamentally expresses, intersects with and is encompassed within broader notions of civil, political and social citizenship, and which are subject to debate (see Lister 1997). Similarly, the issues raised by and for welfare in risk society symbolize and are inseparable from broader economic, political and cultural processes – as we discuss further below. Another reason for our use of 'welfare citizenship' is an attempt to reclaim the word 'welfare' from its increasingly narrow (Americanized) association with social security benefit systems and budgets alone, and restore its reference to a broad gamut of risks, resources and their social distribution.

We begin our discussion of the inter-relationship of risk, citizenship and welfare with a consideration of the basis of traditional solidaristic welfare states, based on systematic risk assessment and posing welfare citizens as citizen-recipients of a rational redistributive state. We then outline the major economic, political and cultural shifts involved in globalization that are argued to undermine and/or cancel the established systems of welfare states' risk calculations and redistributions. Such shifts mean that collective provision has come to be seen as a risk to society itself, and that citizens are posed as citizen-consumers who are increasingly aware of risks, and who can and should take rational and responsible risks in welfare provision, in place of discredited state administrators. Accordingly, we review these arguments and challenges to them. This is followed by an overview of posited frameworks for the future of welfare policy and their implications for social exclusion, as these are informed by and cross-cut with notions of risk and citizenship, and in particular consider ideas of the welfare citizen-participant. At this point, we draw out a series of questions raised by our discussion of risk, citizenship and the issues for welfare, and review the ways in which the following chapters address these. Our discussion, as well as that of a number of contributions to this collection, identifies central issues for, and developments in, welfare in the British context. However, given the arguments about the global and personal nature of risk and the dilemmas for welfare citizenship and provision, the broad issues have a wider relevance, despite the varied political and discursive histories of different national contexts (see, for example, Bussemaker and Voet 1998; Chamberlayne and Rustin 1999).

'Traditional' welfare states: risk sharing and citizen-recipients

The traditional model for extensive or developed welfare states is an institutional nation-state response to coping with unforeseen but broadly predictable consequences, based on actuarial principles and collectively shared rights and responsibilities. It is founded on a solidaristic state-centred response to the meeting of risks encountered within a typical lifecourse on the basis of broad social obligation as part of citizenship, together with the creation of mutual security.

The post-war British welfare state developed in this way, to act to secure risk-free presents and futures through socially collective, state-centred insurance and provision. The welfare risks facing citizens were identified on their behalfs by administrators – Beveridge's five giants: Want, Squalor, Idleness, Ignorance and Disease – as were the steps to be taken to protect and secure welfare citizens on a universal basis from the uncertainties and insecurities inherent in the market. The nature of risk was not part of day-to-day thinking and public debate. Rather, the emphasis was on needs and safety net security. The state was the rational actor, pursuing full employment and calculating the redistribution of resources to promote solidarity between social classes, and to meet the systematic and predictable order of collectively insurable risks encountered by its citizens, whether attached to the labour market or outside. The latter were citizen-recipients, in the sense that welfare citizenship was implicitly based on deference to 'top down' definitions and prescriptions of 'what is best', referred to by John Clarke and Mary Langan as 'attributed need' (1998: 265), and on passive acceptance of policy-makers' and professionals' authority and accredited expertise.

Citizen-recipients had evidence of their welfare citizenship through the rights and responsibilities that accrued to them, and in turn welfare provisions and practices coded the principles and boundaries of citizenship. Indeed, the notion of citizenship, welfare or otherwise, operates simultaneously as a mechanism of inclusion and exclusion (Lister 1997). As Fiona Williams (1989) has pointed out, Beveridge's five giants hid the giants of Sexism and Racism, as well as other forms of discrimination on the basis of age, disability, sexual orientation and so on. While women and Black people and members of other marginalized groups benefited from the general improvements of welfare reforms, at the same time they were excluded from full welfare citizenship covered by universal protection. Caring work was 'domestified', with much policy and provision based on the assumed predominance of the nuclear family form, treating women as dependents of their bread-winning, tenancy-holding husbands (appealing to and reinforcing particular ideas of what constitutes British family). Residency and eligibility qualifications could mean that Black people did not have access to some welfare provisions (embodying particular ideas of national unity). (See Hill Collins (2001) for some kindred discussion of the ways that ideas of family and nation have shaped US welfare citizenship.)

Whatever its strengths and shortcomings, there are arguments that the 'universal' citizenship model of social welfare provision is breaking down. The transition to an unpredictable risk society means that we do not know what the risks are, let alone how to calculate and respond to them, and there are concerns about how to finance these responses (Franklin 1998). Social theorists have posited that challenges to collective social provision through welfare states emanate from two main shifts: (a) a changing international economic, political and cultural context that limits national governments' freedom to pursue independent policies, both economic and social, usually referred to as globalization; and (b) changes in perceptions and experiences of the nature of risk interlinked with a decline in citizens' confidence in, and reliance on, those who administer and provide welfare services. Examples of relevant texts that have been particularly influential in the UK, including in relation to welfare policy developments, include Ulrich Beck (1992, 1999; Beck *et al.* 1994) and Anthony Giddens (1991, 1994, 1998). These shifts mean that governments can no longer easily pursue universalist state-centred economic or social welfare strategies. They also mean that citizens are increasingly aware of risks to their welfare but are sceptical of the abilities of policy-makers and professionals to deal with them, and so turn away from supporting collective state welfare provision to other, more individualized, sources. The nature of welfare citizenship has thus changed as well.

Shifts to economic, political and cultural globalization

Globalization refers to increasing and integrated social processes that are indifferent to national boundaries at economic, political and cultural levels (see authors cited above regarding discussion in this section). Economically, three main and interconnected processes have resulted in an expansion of international competition, and new and flexible labour markets. First, recently developing economies have emerged that can challenge and undercut more established developed economies. Second, international speculative capital has undergone massive growth to the extent that it can now destabilize national currencies and economic policies. Similarly and third, the spread both of multinational corporate companies and of trans-national organizations have also restricted governments' abilities to manage the economy, and in turn influence the scope of welfare policy. Thus economic globalization means, for example, that levels of un-, under- or sub-employment are increasingly outside national governments' control and they are limited in their ability to promote social equality (should they have this as an aim). Furthermore, economic developments towards global consumption can increase people's sense of themselves as consumers, including consumers of welfare – an issue we return to below.

Interconnected with economic shifts is globalization in formal political structures, whereby state sovereignty and centralized structures are weakened and shrinking. There is a transition from a nation-state to a cosmopolitan world order, and the concept of political community changes. Transnational political regimes have developed and the nation-state's control of the remit or content of national citizenship and state action can be shaped and overridden by international jurisdictions such as the International Court of Justice and the Human Rights Charter, and by supranational political bodies such as the expanding European Union. Political globalization creates the space for an institutionalized individualization of rights, including to welfare, independent of nationality – it bypasses nations and states to address individuals directly, raising the issue of multiple citizenship on several political levels and with the potential for envisaging a status of world or global citizenship.[3]

Culturally, globalization is furthered through instant communication and rapid developments in information technologies. While this aspect of globalization can, on the one hand, evidence a convergence in culture, lifestyle and values (for example, the 'Coca Cola generation'), on the other hand, it can equally give people greater awareness, knowledge of and access to a diversity of lifestyles, and access to a variety of viewpoints and information (the 'cosmopolitan gaze' in Beck's (2000) terms). 'Natural' gendered divisions of labour and sexual orientation, and racialized hierarchies, for example, are open to question. This makes the claim to authoritative knowledge about 'what is good for' citizens and welfare users on the part of policy-makers and practitioners that is implicit in traditional 'top-down' state welfare systems, subject to questioning and critical evaluation by those very welfare citizens. Expert knowledge becomes demystified. People are increasingly aware that opinions can be divided and contested amongst experts, and that there is a diversity of experts, so that they can no longer rely on a single authoritative guidance and action. 'Givens' are dissolved and transformed into choices amongst a number of courses, which entails making decisions. These decisions are presupposed by and subject to risk – uncertainty creates their being taken and there is uncertainty about their outcomes.

Questioning welfare provision: perceptions of risk and the rational citizen-consumer

The traditional remit of welfare states and the risks that they were developed to deal with were understood as the outcome of 'natural' forces, such as birth, sickness, old age and death, or as similarly 'natural' external human interventions, such as accidents and happenstance. However, social theorists of the 'risk society' argue that social and individual perceptions of uncertainty and insecurity in the 'second age of modernity' (Beck 1999, 2000) now encompass awareness that technological, economic or social interventions can generate unpredictable side effects or consequences. These then form new risks, both in the short and long terms. Risk is regarded as pervasive and central in late modernity, on both personal and global levels. The problems that welfare citizens face in their everyday lives are now seen as being influenced by global economic, technological and social forces that are both incalculable and beyond the control of governments, or at least within their control only in a limited sense. In itself this challenges the security of welfare citizenship. As described above, labour markets are at the mercy of extra-national developments and the decisions of multinational corporations, and the introduction of new technologies brings job insecurity for sections of the labour force.

The growths in life expectancy and in diversity of family forms (lone mother-hood, cohabitation, step, non-heterosexual and so on) mean that treating these as collective risks has become too large an economic burden. Moreover, women's employment has increased over the last decades, further increasing the collective welfare burden. The traditional 'invisible' informal underpinnings of welfare state provision, whereby women, supported by a male breadwinner, cared for older and disabled people, and for their own children, in the domestic sphere, is no longer unquestioningly available. Such disruptions to traditional and predictable life-courses mean that it has become more difficult and less feasible for welfare states to offer collective social protection against risks.

But it is not just that traditional state-centred methods of welfare provision may no longer be able to cope, it is said, but that citizens perceive the welfare risks to which they are potentially subject as more pressing and the future as more uncertain. The awareness and apprehension of risk and insecurity permeates society (although, as Peter Taylor-Gooby (2000a) has argued, for some social groups, such as the middle classes, this is to a much greater extent than the actual welfare risks they face themselves). Furthermore, as noted earlier, citizens have far less trust in received wisdoms and the state as a welfare provider that can deal in any adequate way with these current and future uncertainties. Citizens' confidence in the power of authoritative administration to plan for and control economic and social life, and accredited professionals' abilities to meet their individual needs, is undermined. Politicians and professionals are increasingly seen as having their own interests at heart (votes, power, budgets, etc.), rather than the welfare needs of citizens.

Citizens have thus become critical of the role of government in welfare provision, and there has been a growth in social and lifestyle pressure groups and self-help movements, forming new active welfare citizenship identities (Eyerman and Jamison 1991; Touraine 1981; Williams 1989, 1999). Groups constructed as outside of, or marginalized by, traditional notions of citizenship and its civil, political and social rights on the basis of gender, ethnicity, sexuality and disability, no longer accept this top–down imposition. They challenge not just access to citizenship but the basis of it, extending the very constitution of welfare citizenship. Such groups and movements have also been instrumental in highlighting new social risks, such as domestic violence and child abuse, homophobia, and racial violence and discrimination.

The traditional version of the welfare state is also under attack from both the New Right and Third Way political proponents, who argue that the state's proper role should now be the management of risk, rather than collective social provision, and that citizens are rational welfare-consumers.

The New Right perceives the welfare state, not as a source of protection from insecurity and uncertainty, but rather as a source of economic, moral and cultural risk generation in itself. It poses risks to entrepreneurship and initiative, and to work incentives and economic competitiveness, and concomitant risks of dependency and an underclass, and of inefficient and expensive public sector services (for example, Green 1998, 1999; and see discussion by Culpitt 1999). The institution introduced to mitigate risks to citizens' welfare has generated the risk of social breakdown. Fundamentally, citizens are regarded as self-interested individuals who make rational choices after assessing their personal risks, weighing up the costs and benefits of courses of action available to them, and then pursuing the one that maximizes their personal benefit and limits the costs to them. Within this view of life, the logic of collective responsibility and provision is anti-rational, inappropriate and harmful. People will not contribute towards collective efforts to realize social profits if they can achieve such profits without participating. The provision of 'generous' welfare benefits and services has thus perversely altered the proper balance between citizenship rights and obligations (stressing the former over the latter), and affected the parameters for rational decision-making. It has enabled, for example, men to live without undertaking paid work, mothers to bring up children without fathers, and children to evade responsibility for their elderly parents. Welfare rights turned citizens into passive claimants with no obligations, and the resultant 'welfare dependency' has become a perverse form of social inclusion.

In addition, it is argued that because the welfare state has led to 'scrounging', 'good' citizens no longer identify with a wider common welfare 'community', and are less prepared to finance collective state-centred provision through taxes. The private sector, with its substantial resources and individualized customer ethos, is seen as more satisfactory in both providing choice and avoiding dependency culture. The charitable and voluntary sector will provide for those who are unable to purchase their own welfare provisions (Green 1993).

Risk theorists can also pose people as rational choice-makers, including in relation to welfare provision. (See Culpitt (1999) for a broader discussion of risk theorists in relation to social welfare policy.) Both Ulrich Beck and Anthony Giddens, for example, argue that individualization is associated with risk society, whereby risk perception and protection is focused in and on the dimension of the individual rather than a given, communal collectivity and hierarchy. Both regard the individual in a risk society as a creative agent. However, Beck (1996, 2000) sees the individualization process as an automatic reflex-like epistemological paradigm shift beyond rational choice and towards indistinctness and ambivalence, not merely an increase in the significance of knowledge and reflection. In contrast, Giddens (1991, 1994, 1998) tends to focus on the latter.

Giddens stresses a more rational human agency within a deliberately formulated and pursued 'Third Way' state political paradigm 'beyond left and right' in order to manage risk. Citizens feel themselves responsible for 'building their own biography', assessing and appraising their options and planning and pursuing their own lifestyles. They are more inclined to live their lives as an active self-fulfilment project than to follow traditional prescriptions and paths, given their awareness that a diversity of lifestyles and values is available to them and their questioning of authoritative expertise. They formulate strategies to meet their own welfare as they define it. People are no longer citizen-recipients but increasingly see themselves as, and feel the need to be, citizen-consumers. They are preoccupied by and identify with risk and uncertainty, defining and taking responsibility for their own welfare and making choices about how best and from what source to meet it, entailing a new balance between individual and collective rights and responsibilities. The welfare state should focus on 'positive welfare' and be concerned with shaping the environment for citizens to be and behave as 'responsible risk-takers' (Giddens 1998: 100, 116).

New Right and Third Way explicit or implicit assumptions and depictions of autonomous rational citizen-consumers have been challenged (for example, Duncan and Edwards 1999; Taylor-Gooby 1998, 2000a and b; Taylor-Gooby *et al.* 1999; Sevenhuijsen 2000). Several issues are pertinent to our discussion here. People perceive and respond to risks across a wide range of aspects of their lives from the particular social context in which they are embedded, with different groups both perceiving their situation, and having the capacity to act, in different, and in unequal, ways. Furthermore, they are embedded in situated relationships and networks of care-giving and receiving, which are subject to gendered inequalities, but care work is not recognized as part of citizenship rights and responsibilities in the same way as paid work. In relation to current formal welfare citizenship, the private sector is not necessarily a good alternative for the citizen-consumer. It is as much subject to the economic and cultural changes and pressures affecting welfare provision as is the state provider. Moreover, citizens can still support state responsibility for meeting common welfare needs and interests, even given its shortcoming and perceptions of individual responsibility, and can mistrust alternative welfare providers.

Yet, constraints in the universal coverage provided by the welfare state promoted by the New Right and Third Way analysts in themselves lead to apprehension that the major mechanism for managing risk and insecurity is no longer sufficient or available, and those who are able to will purchase private services to meet their needs (Taylor-Gooby 2000a). Indeed, a sense of uncertainty and anxiety is heightened by this very ability to choose – the risk of making a wrong choice. As discussed further below, given the evidence from several chapters in this collection, there is also a similar argument to be made that the current operation of the British welfare state benefit and service provisions can exacerbate groups of citizens' feelings of uncertainty and risk.

There are also further and significant difficulties, in terms of social exclusion, in accepting the inevitability of, or actively pursuing, a welfare citizen-consumer model of provision in 'risk society'.

W(h)ither the welfare state?: social exclusion and the citizen-participant

Social exclusion has become a topic of much political and academic debate, and represents a recent shift from stated concerns about an 'underclass' towards a notion of 'social exclusion'. Both of these terms can be seen as 'political artefacts' in the sense that they are the creation of political and discursive processes (Chamberlayne 1997). The socially excluded are constructed as categories of people, such as lone mothers, the long-term unemployed and unqualified youth, and disabled, older and minority ethnic people. These groups are deemed to be outwith the contemporary mainstream of economic and cultural life and of full citizenship through their reliance on welfare benefits. As Ruth Levitas (1996) has pointed out, such a notion posits a two-part society – the excluded and the included. It conflates social exclusion with exclusion from the labour market, erasing from view inequalities within the 'included', such as those who are in low paid insecure employment. It also devalues the unpaid care work carried out principally by women. Several contributions to this book are concerned with such issues, in particular focusing on those on the margins of 'inclusion' and subject to the risk of exclusion.

Posited frameworks for welfare policy, as these cross-cut with notions of citizenship and are underpinned by understandings of risk, thus have particular implications for social exclusion and attempts to mould citizens' behaviour so as to avoid it. Analyses of 'risk society' and the concomitant portrayal of a turning away from collective social provision through the welfare state, have led to debates about the direction of UK welfare policies, which have become more marked in recent decades. Several trajectories that can overlap at various points can be identified (see, for example, Beck 2000; Etzioni 1995; Franklin 1998; Giddens 1994, 1998; Lister 1997; Selbourne 1994; Taylor-Gooby *et al.* 1999; Williams 1999).

One possibility is that policies can remain static. This can be posited on two bases. First, in a risk society, it can be argued that all attempts at reformulation in themselves bear the seeds of new and more difficult risks. Second, alternatively or additionally, stasis can be seen as an attempt to preserve and strengthen the traditional institutions and relationships that once served citizens well (or at least White male breadwinner citizens), and provided a secure backdrop to national economic and social life. This 'more of the same' approach can also involve a focus on the state intervening to ensure that people's behaviour fits with tradition, with citizenship eligibility rights for certain publicly funded entitlements conditional on individuals conforming to laid down patterns, and the profiling of risks to prevent their occurrence. The state remains the rational actor and welfare citizens continue to be citizen-recipients. With a static approach to narrow institutional social policy concerns along traditional lines, new circumstances and risks will not be addressed. Those groups previously excluded will remain so, including those who care within the domestic sphere, and they and other groups affected by the new risks will be placed outside of welfare citizenship.

Alternatively, policies can enthusiastically pursue retrenchment. Here, the welfare remit of the state is seen as concerned with 'investing' in society, and policies are pursued that are designed to enhance national competitiveness in a global labour market and/or are intended to promote education and training for a flexible and highly skilled labour force. Redistributive policies are abandoned. Again, there can be a focus on state intervention to modify people's behaviour, here to reduce risky actions rather than providing services to deal with the outcomes of those actions. The service providers, in private and voluntary sectors, then undertake the profiling of risks and their management. The state is only justified in providing a discriminatory residual and minimal 'safety net', with the driving force of welfare provision being the rational citizen-consumer. With retrenchment even many 'old' risks will be placed outside socially collective, state-centred provision, placing particular groups subject to both old and new risks outside of welfare citizenship.

Both New Right and Third Way policy adherents advocate such retrenchment, but the latter can also draw on ideas about states attempting to understand and work with the process of change, focusing on creating new parameters for, and choices in, welfare policies through restructuring. In this formulation, political frameworks are complemented by democratic dialogue outside state institutions that enables a diversity of interests to negotiate the meeting of welfare needs. For some, this dialogue can form the basis for an inclusive but differentiated universalism in citizenship. However, such restructuring notions (in Third Way prescriptions) can just as easily shade into welfare consumerism and retrenchment, with the state providing the regulative framework and ensuring information provision so that citizen-consumers can go into the marketplace to meet their own needs, as they can lead to a new state-centred social collective welfare consensus. The welfare citizenship arguments that can be used to support and justify the case for collective social support can be turned around to advocate individualistic welfare consumers' rights to choice. With a stress on responsible risk taking in addressing new social welfare risks, and a decline in confidence in the expertise of policy-makers and professionals, those who can afford it will tend to search outside of the state welfare systems for ensuring security and welfare. Those who rely on these systems can then be disadvantaged and socially marginalized.

In a risk society critique can become democratized. Anthony Giddens' (1998) variant of the citizen-consumer replaces the authority of government and professionals with an individualized citizen-participant. As Selma Sevenhuijsen (2000) has pointed out however, this also draws on an essentially conservative philosophy, including an assumed opposition between the independent individual and social ties and collectivity, and a reification of labour market participation as the paradigm for citizenship. In contrast, she calls for welfare citizenship to be guided by a feminist ethic of care that acknowledges individuals as existing through and situated within relational ties, addresses inequalities in the distribution of paid work and of informal care giving and receiving, and respects difference as part of equality (Sevenhuijsen 1998, 2000). Indeed positing a new framework for a welfare state is a quest for many on the radical and feminist left. This framework is rooted in commitment to universal coverage and social redistribution, and espousal of a welfare citizenship that recognizes people's own definitions of their diversity and particularity, not only inequalities in society at large, thus encompassing a broader notion of the welfare citizen-participant. Fiona Williams (1999), for example, has proposed key 'good enough' principles for the reordering of the social relations of welfare: interdependence, care, intimacy, bodily integrity, identity, transnational welfare and voice. These principles build on notions of welfare citizenship as social groups defining risks to their welfare and actively participating in the democratic organization of a redistributive welfare state. (See also Lister (1997) for a move towards transcending gender equality and difference debates and other binaries in relation to citizenship in its broad sense.)

Ulrich Beck (2000) optimistically identifies the paradigm shifts that such a restructuring of the basis of welfare states would entail as part of the opportunity of a risk society. Although his work may be subject to the criticism of dichotomous assumptions, such as between the individual and the communal, and rights and responsibilities, he nonetheless poses risk societies as moving towards combining the apparently mutually exclusive, and as based on questions that can be answered differently. It is to such questions as they relate to particularistic intersections of risk, citizenship and welfare that we now turn.

Risk and citizenship: questions for welfare

Several sets of questions concerning welfare collectivity, redistribution, social practice and provision arise from our review of the issues surrounding welfare, risk and citizenship. These include:

- Can collective values and provision be maintained in the context of increasing economic, political and cultural change that has much to do with globalization? What would be the basis for this? Is it possible for governments to develop policies that nurture collective values in the face of individualization? Is it in the interests of market capitalism to do this?
- In a context of large and rapid changes in the ways in which citizens live, work and relate to each other, can traditional welfare state concerns with redistribution be maintained? If risks of various sorts are not equally distributed, with some social groups being considerably more vulnerable to welfare risks than others, is there any future for a risk-pooling approach? If social inequalities persist, how does this leave a policy context where national governments are becoming progressively less powerful, not only because citizens have less confidence in them, but also because of supranational pressures?
- Does increasing access to lifestyle diversity amongst citizens lead to the replacement of traditional moral values? What are the risks associated with new values – are they viewed as opportunities or as threats? Are we witnessing the birth of new kinds of moral welfare collectivism and citizen-participation, with social and cultural diversity rather than sameness as its basis? Are we also seeing an increase in local collectivism and risk-taking? Or does the erosion of traditional moral values lead to dependency and social exclusion?

- As part of the process of individualization people are said to be increasingly assuming that the problems facing them are only solvable via their own actions. If part of a risk society is a growing view that the state cannot provide welfare solutions and also that it should not, what is the role of social policy in dealing with uncertainty? Although responsible risk-taking may be feasible and indeed welcome for some, where does that leave those citizens who cannot or will not self-manage risks to their welfare? In the face of notions of social exclusion, and of negative and pathologizing government rhetoric about 'welfare dependency', what are the implications for the relationship between citizen-recipients and governments?

- Governments in late modernity may wish to work with individualization and encourage the emergence of citizen-consumers in terms of choice and autonomy in relation to the self-management of welfare. What does this mean for governments' ability to manage citizens' welfare risk-taking in relation to the ways in which they seek to provide for themselves? With individualization, will citizens' efforts to avoid social exclusion include informal, or even illegal, methods of provision?

- What does the relationship between risk management and risk assessment mean for welfare citizenship? Can needs-based assessment of citizen-recipients coexist with rights-based notions of the citizen-consumer and/or dialogic notions of citizen-participants in welfare provision? Can professional expertise mix with responsible risk-taking and individualization? Can governments take account of a diversity of welfare citizenships?

These questions variously underpin and inform the contributions to this edited collection. We start with chapters that deal with broad and general issues, moving on to those that focus on specific policies and ending with chapters that deal with practice.

In Chapter 2, Paul Spicker issues a challenge to sociological perspectives on risk, as he sees them. Instead of taking risk as central, as is the case in analyses of 'risk society', he sees risk as one element of a generic category of insecurity, examining the ways in which systems of social protection can respond to these different forms of insecurity. The issues that are raised by a consideration of the different forms of insecurity are wider, he concludes, than issues of income and wealth. Spicker emphasizes the need for systems of social protection to take on board issues such as autonomy and the protection of a person's lifestyle. This clearly takes us beyond the passive citizen-recipient of the post-war era.

Zsuzsa Ferge explores the concept of the social contract between government and citizens in the context of globalization and market capitalism in Chapter 3. Her perspective is a refreshing one, since she argues that a 'messy' relationship between government and citizens is far from being a problem. In making this statement, Ferge is arguing for diversity, meaning that less powerful social groups will have a better chance of getting access to resources. This is unlike the traditional approaches to welfare that have favoured either residualism, market solutions, reciprocity or social rights. Ferge argues that a combination of these is more appropriate for the social and political context in which we find ourselves at the beginning of the twenty-first century. Conceptual clarity is a legitimate analytical exercise, but reality is different. Human relations are complex and the relations between citizens and governments are similarly complex. A combination of traditions is more likely to respond in a fair and dignified way to this complexity and diversity.

In Chapter 4, a broad definition of citizenship is advocated by Jeffrey Weeks, who argues for the encompassing of various forms of diversity, including sexuality. This perspective impinges closely on the issue of social order, since traditional forms of morality are questioned in a fundamental way. Furthermore, the widening of the ambit of citizenship recognizes the shifting relationships between men and women, men and men, women and women to a situation where the egalitarian relationship is increasingly a goal (although not necessarily one that is always realized). For Weeks, the twin developments of the undermining of traditional moral values and the transformation of intimate relations are themselves located in the rapid economic, social and cultural changes which are taking place on a global scale. New moral values have, Weeks argues, reasserted collective values in the form of a new culture of responsibility for others. The new morality has also created autonomy through the choices that many people have to make in order to find meaningful ways of living together. For some this is a threat, for others this is an opportunity.

Also seeking to widen the definition of citizenship, in Chapter 5 Jan Pahl addresses a particular sort of citizenship that covers access to financial products and services. She looks at both the macro aspect of differential access to financial services, as well as the micro aspect of individuals' access to such services within families. Full citizenship, she argues, should include full access to financial services, in view of its impact on financial welfare and it should be an attribute of the individual and not of the household in which s/he lives. Recent changes have taken place in the use of credit cards and banking and Pahl examines the implications for social policy of these changes, in the light of research into financial arrangements within families. Pahl shows that the allocation of money within the family continues to show inequalities between women and men. Men have more knowledge of and access to new ways of controlling finances, implying unequal access to citizenship within the household. For Pahl, the policy implications are twofold: first, citizen-consumers need to have access to transparent information about financial services and this has implications for the regulation of financial services by governments. Second, citizen-consumers need to have wider access to banking and credit if they are not to suffer financial and social exclusion. This implies that governments should lift restrictions that prevent people from taking control of their finances through local, collective action.

In Chapter 6, Peter Taylor-Gooby pursues theoretical debates about gender, class and inequality, asking whether the pursuit of both class and gender egalitarianism can be sustained in modern social policy without prejudicing one or the other.

Before presenting evidence to show that the achievement of gender equality in wages would not be at the expense of an increase in social class inequalities, Taylor-Gooby reviews the social and economic developments that provide a context for his analysis. He concludes that gender and class inequalities must be tackled at the same time through social policy, since unintended consequences might come about if one was tackled at the expense of the other. Focusing particularly on the UK, Taylor-Gooby implies that the 'Third Way' social policy approach of New Labour has the potential to abandon the traditional left concern with class inequality and he points out that there may well be electoral implications of this. The reason for New Labour's reduced focus on class based inequalities is their assumption that welfare policy is subject to individualization. This is implicit in New Labour's emphasis on individual opportunity and its reduction of interest in outcomes, an Old Labour concern. Taylor-Gooby argues that the New Labour emphasis on equality of opportunity will simply sustain current patterns of household inequality. Inequalities between households will not be tackled without an emphasis on equality of outcome. Both policy and analysis need to take account of the intersecting and multivariate nature of disadvantage.

Ruth Lister similarly addresses particularly pertinent issues for the UK's policy context in Chapter 7. Traditional (Old Labour) debates about the adequacy of benefit levels and about structural aspects of welfare cannot be ignored, as New Labour appears to be doing in its shift from an equality agenda to the promotion of opportunity through paid work. If there is little debate on these issues, Lister argues, a large number of people will experience increasing financial and social insecurity, with implications for their status as citizens. Lister asserts strongly that the reality of New Labour's policies differs considerably from its rhetoric (which is in itself inconsistent). New Labour runs the risk of abandoning principles of social justice, although its rhetoric denies this. It has continued the New Right rhetoric on the risks to society posed by a 'dependency culture' and this has the potential to alienate many service users, with the attendant risk of a growing number of citizens becoming alienated from government. Redistribution still exists, but redistribution of resources has given way to redistribution of opportunity, with a clear emphasis on paid work. Lister concludes that the net effect of New Labour's policies will be greater financial insecurity and consequently a fracturing of social citizenship.

In Chapter 8, using the concept of a risk economy, David Abbott and Deborah Quilgars make the point that the insecurity generated by flexible labour markets has taken place at the same time as a shrinking of the welfare safety net. But risk is not equally distributed across social classes. Since some groups are able to buy freedom from risk, risks echo the inequalities of class society. Abbott and Quilgars ask whether people in poverty plan for the future, including the risk of social exclusion through unemployment. They conclude that welfare provided by the private sector cannot cope with the consequences of risky labour markets. Furthermore, public policy changes based on rational choice theory are questionable. Rational choice theory says that future risks are calculable, but the evidence from Abbott and Quilgars is that they are not, as Taylor-Gooby (2000b) has also concluded. In addition, their research revealed little faith amongst their research subjects that state-provided welfare could be a sufficiently generous backstop in the event of unemployment, together with an acceptance that welfare was changing and that self-provision was inevitable. Both the traditional 'safety net' system and its citizen-recipients were perceived in an increasingly negative light.

In Chapter 9, Kathryn Ellis and Ann Davis examine the different sorts of risk assessment used within community care by policy-makers, professionals and service users. They explore risk assessment theoretically, largely from a Foucauldian point of view, and empirically through a three-way comparison of different approaches to risk assessment. As the welfare state restructured in the 1980s, so community care policies were developed, principally for economic reasons, in order to minimize the costs of dependency. The means of doing this was to develop risk-based prioritization criteria, which allowed professionals to manage care by first scrutinizing the needs of citizen-recipient users and subsequently interrogating their carers in order to set up economically efficient packages of care. The implication here is that the assessed needs would not necessarily be met in their entirety by the state and that the remainder would have to be met by users' carers. An aspect of this restructured approach was the pre-scription of needs by generic social worker teams, whereby 'risk/needs matrices' set out prescribed criteria for the assessment of priorities. Thus the definition of needs was circumscribed in advance of the assessment, so that assessed needs could be allocated to the predetermined and 'expert' categories of risk. A three-way comparison of different approaches to risk assessment by generic social worker teams, hospital teams and teams which specialized in particular sorts of disability showed that only the latter viewed risk in a non-defensive way by collaborating with citizen-participant users in balancing both positive and negative outcomes of risk.

In their examination of an informal labour market in South London, David Smith and John Macnicol address issues of autonomy and citizenship in Chapter 10. The 'survival strategies' of people faced with economic risk are explored, in a context of the economic transformations that have affected advanced industrialized economies over the past quarter-century. Labour market uncertainty affects different social groups differently, but even amongst those hardest hit by labour market uncertainty, agency and control over their own lives were strongly desired. Smith and Macnicol make the important point, as Beck (1992) does, that as the traditional social class structure has become increasingly diversified, so it has been replaced by patterns of inequality that are based on the ability to buy privatized welfare. Their research reveals a form of entrepreneurial risk-taking (albeit illegal) that yields undeclared income, which is in turn underpinned by the benefit system. The people studied here were very far from regarding themselves as an 'underclass' or victims and were seeking to avoid social exclusion. Indeed, from this perspective, although questionable from the point of view of traditional moral values, uncertainty could be viewed as positive since it provides opportunities.

In our final chapter, written from the perspective of economics, Barbara Jones and Bob Miller take the view that social capital, in the sense of mutual trust, knowledge, networks and community, has an increasingly urgent need to be nurtured. This is because of capitalism's accelerating 'cycles of destruction' which counteract the development and preservation of collective values. Focusing specifically on the skills and knowledge of people working in information and communication technologies (ICT), Jones and Miller trace the consequences for social capital of cycles of disinvestment. They conclude that governments need to consider how to encourage individuals to invest in social capital, such that social networks are restored. If social capital is irretrievably lost, then there is a need to consider how welfare needs and risks previously met and managed with 'communities' can be provided for, either through the market or the state.

The specific issues explored in many of the chapters in this collection are not necessarily 'new' risks and aspects of welfare citizenship. Where we think that we have covered new ground is in our selection of issues that exemplify our typology of different types of welfare citizenship as these identify and respond to risk. The typology that we have used in this introductory chapter – the citizen-recipient, the citizen-consumer and the citizen-participant – can be located in different ideological contexts, although the three categories of citizenship should not be seen as leading on neatly from one to the other in a linear way. Rather, they are types that overlap and they may even exist coterminously, both in a macro sense within the nation-state and globally, as well as in a micro sense within families. This implies the coexistence (possibly not particularly harmonious) of different types of welfare citizenship. A major challenge for governments must be how to devise policies that address, possibly simultaneously, these types of welfare citizenship. We are at a point of great historical interest, when rapid changes are taking place in the relationship between governments and citizens. This collection adds to the debates on risk and citizenship as these relate to welfare, by laying out policy and practice in a range of different social policy contexts in order to put flesh on this changing relationship.

Notes

1 We would like to thank Jane Franklin for helpful comments on an earlier version of this chapter.
2 The topics addressed are by no means comprehensive in terms of welfare citizenship and risk issues; education and several aspects of health care, for example, are not addressed. In addition, issues of race/ethnicity feature less than we are comfortable with, despite the editorial intention not to marginalize ethnicity or gender by including separate chapters on these issues but to encourage all authors to take account of them.
3 Although retaining a notion of citizenship, with its connotations of boundaries and outsiders as well as inclusion, under a global all-encompassing coverage, seems rather incongruous.

References

Beck, U. (1992) *Risk Society: Towards a New Modernity*, London: Sage.

—— (1996) 'Risk society and the provident state', in S. Lash, B. Szerszynski and B. Wynne (eds) *Risk, Environment and Modernity*, London: Sage.

—— (1999) *World Risk Society*, Cambridge: Polity Press.

—— (2000) 'The cosmopolitan perspective: sociology of the second age of modernity', *British Journal of Sociology*, 51(2): 79–105.

Beck, U., Giddens, A. and Lash, S. (1994) *Reflexive Modernisation*, Cambridge: Polity Press.

Bussemaker, J. and Voet, R. (eds) (1998) *Critical Social Policy Special Issue: Vocabularies of Citizenship and Gender*, 18:3.

Chamberlayne, P. (1997) *Social Exclusion in Comparative Perspective*, SOSTRIS Working Paper No. 1, University of East London.

Chamberlayne, P. and Rustin, M. (1999) *From Biography to Social Policy, Final Report of the Social Strategies in Risk Societies Project*, SOSTRIS Working Paper No. 9, University of East London.

Clarke, J. and Langan, M. (1998) 'Review', in M. Langan (ed.) *Welfare: Needs, Rights and Risks*, Milton Keynes: Open University Press.

Culpitt, I. (1999) *Social Policy and Risk*, London: Sage.

Duncan, S. and Edwards, R. (1999) *Lone Mothers, Paid Work and Gendered Moral Rationalities*, Basingstoke: Macmillan.

Etzioni, A. (1995) *The Spirit of Community: Rights and Responsibilities and the Communitarian Agenda*, London: HarperCollins.

Eyerman, R. and Jamison, A. (1991) *Social Movements: A Cognitive Approach*, Cambridge: Polity Press.

Franklin, J. (ed.) (1998) *The Politics of Risk Society*, Cambridge: Polity Press.

Giddens, A. (1991) *Modernity and Self-Identity: Self and Society in the Late Modern Age*, Cambridge: Polity Press.

—— (1994) *Beyond Left and Right*, Cambridge: Polity Press.

—— (1998) *The Third Way: The Renewal of Social Democracy*, Cambridge: Polity Press.

Hill Collins, P. (2001) 'Like one of the family: race, ethnicity and the paradox of US national identity', *Ethnic and Racial Studies*, 24(1): 3–28.

Green, D. (1993) *Reinventing Civil Society: The Rediscovery of Welfare Without Politics*, London: Institute for Economic Affairs.

—— (1998) *Benefit Dependency: How Welfare Undermines Independence*, London: Institute for Economic Affairs.

—— (1999) *An End to Welfare Rights: The Rediscovery of Independence*, London: Institute for Economic Affairs.

Levitas, R. (1996) 'The concept of social exclusion and the new Durkheiman legacy', *Critical Social Policy*, 16(1): 5–20.

Lister, R. (1997) *Citizenship: Feminist Perspectives*, Basingstoke: Macmillan.

Selbourne, D. (1994) *The Principle of Duty*, London: Sinclair Stevenson.

Sevenhuijsen, S. (1998) *Citizenship and the Ethics of Care: Feminist Considerations on Justice, Morality and Politics*, London: Routledge.

—— (2000) 'Caring in the Third Way: the relation between obligation, responsibility and care in Third Way discourse', *Critical Social Policy* 20(1): 5–37.

Taylor-Gooby, P. (ed.) (1998) *Choice and Public Policy*, Basingstoke: Macmillan.

—— (ed.) (2000a) *Risk, Trust and Welfare*, Basingstoke: Macmillan.

—— (2000b) 'Risk, contingency and the Third Way: evidence from BHPS and qualitative studies', Social Policy Association Annual Conference, *Futures of Social Policy and Practice?*', University of Surrey Roehampton, July.

Taylor-Gooby, P., Dean, H., Munro, M. and Parker, G. (1999) 'Risk and the welfare state', *British Journal of Sociology* 50(2): 177–94.

Touraine, A. (1981) *The Voice and the Eye: An Analysis of Social Movements*, Cambridge: Cambridge University Press.

Williams, F. (1989) *Social Policy: A Critical Introduction. Issues of Race, Gender and Class*, Cambridge: Polity Press.

—— (1999) 'Good enough principles for welfare', *Journal of Social Policy* 28(4): 667–87.

Chapter 2

Social insecurity and social protection

Paul Spicker

The image of 'insecurity' which occurs in current sociological literature begins from a series of premises which many in the field of social policy would find difficult to accept. Giddens suggests that we are in a 'post scarcity' society, and that in the condition of post scarcity our attention has been focused on risks, real or imagined. He writes:

> The welfare state cannot survive in its existing form . . . the current problems of the welfare state should not be seen as a fiscal crisis but one of the management of risk.
>
> (Giddens 1994: 174)

This reflects the influence of Ulrich Beck, whose fashionable 'risk society' (Beck, 1992) conjures a picture of a society (uncannily like parts of Germany) where people have been sensitized to risk because they have no more serious problems to contend with. Beck describes an atomized society, where individuals have been deracinated:

> 'Individualisation' means, first, the disembedding of industrial-society ways of life and, secondly, the re-embedding of new ones, in which the individuals must produce, stage and cobble together their biographies themselves. . . . Both – disembedding and re-embedding – do not occur by chance, nor individually, nor voluntarily, nor through diverse types of historical conditions, but rather all at once and under the general conditions of the welfare state in advanced industrial society.
>
> (Beck 1997: 95)

This is an old marxist chestnut, tied to the idea that capitalism replaced the cosy social relationships of feudalism with a cash nexus. If one accepts that it is true, the subsequent development of solidarity, social protection and the welfare state (see Baldwin 1990) becomes baffling. As for Beck's contention that insecurity is increasing, Steuer is scathing:

To provide counter examples to Professor Beck's image of the predictable past and the risky present is embarrassing because it is like the proverbial activity of shooting fish in a barrel. We have world wars to draw on, massive flu epidemics, and depressions with widespread economic uncertainty. Agricultural production, which involved larger numbers of mankind in the past, is always risky. . . . For most individuals in most parts of the world the chances at birth of dying before the age of 70 are lower today compared to 100 years ago.

(Steuer, 1998: 16)

A fuller critical discussion of these positions can be found in *Social policy in a changing society* (Mullard and Spicker 1998). There are real problems relating to insecurity, but this is not the way to identify them. This chapter looks at the issues of risk and insecurity, and examines the ways in which systems of social protection can respond to those risks.

Insecurity: five concepts

Insecurity, like many words in popular use, has a wide range of meanings, and I do not plan to look at all of them. Several different concepts of insecurity exist side by side in social policy. They include, for example, material, social, economic, financial, psychological and existential insecurity; they may be applied distinctly in a range of fields, including health, wealth, housing and personal autonomy. This chapter is mainly concerned with issues of material and social insecurity, as opposed to psychological insecurity or existential panic. I have selected five main concepts, partly because they seem most directly relevant to social policy, and partly because, taken together, they address the range of issues I wanted to discuss.

Lack of basic security

The first sense in which the idea of insecurity might be used is closely allied to poverty. Wresinski identified a 'lack of basic security' as

the absence of one or more factors that enable individuals and families to assume basic responsibilities and to enjoy fundamental rights . . . chronic poverty results when the lack of basic security simultaneously affects several aspects of people's lives, when it is prolonged, and when it seriously compromises people's chances of regaining their rights and of resuming their responsibilities in the foreseeable future.

(Wresinski Report of the Economic and Social Council of France 1987, cited in Duffy 1995: 35)

This concept is partly material, and partly social. The root of insecurity is the lack of resources, which means that each part of a person's social life is compromised by the limitations this places on each person's capacity. The link between poverty and lack of resources is indirect; poverty, by this account, is a result of the inability to participate in society, and the inability to participate the result of lack of resources.

The connections here are not very clearly worked out, but they are plausible. There are two key points. First, although insecurity can be based in material circumstances, it is defined in social terms. Poor people are likely to be insecure, because the range of positive options open to the poor is limited, and the range of negative options is wide, and the potential to limit damage from negative outcomes is restricted. But there are cases in which poor people are not insecure, and they are defined by the poor person's social position: in a caste society, for example, people of low caste are guaranteed certain occupations (Leach 1960). It is the social position, then, which defines the level of security, not the poverty itself.

Second, insecurity is understood in terms of rights and responsibilities. Rights and responsibilities are central to a place in society, and a place in society is necessary for security. This sounds strange at first, because often security seems to depend on other factors – for example, subsistence farmers in developing countries depend on the weather. Drèze and Sen dispute this, persuasively. They take a strongly relational view of famine, viewing it as the result, not of lack of food, but of lack of entitlement to the food which is otherwise available. The rights of poor people are central to their security; Drèze and Sen argue that political pluralism plays an important part in protecting the position of the poor, and there has never been a famine in a democracy (Drèze and Sen 1989).

Social protection against a lack of basic security is achieved primarily by the provision of a basic foundation of services, and (Drèze and Sen argue) by the provision of basic rights, which are a precondition for protection. These rights have to be general, in the sense of being available to the whole population. Many systems rely primarily on particular rights to provide social protection – that is, individualized rights which are earned through contributions or work-record. Social protection in these circumstances cannot effectively depend on this principle, because particular rights presuppose the ability to contribute.

Risk

The second sense of insecurity is concerned with certain contingencies – things that may happen. Certain eventualities are unpredictable. People know they will die, but they do not know when. They may be disabled, or unemployed or suffer accidents. These contingencies do not apply to everyone, but many if not most people are liable to them, which implies both an element of insecurity and a need for protection.

The area which is outlined here is a different area of concern from the issue currently being dealt with by the sociology of risk. The sociology of risk has focused as much on general doubts about society – environmental concerns and the scope of human action – as on issues relating to insecurity. This is important because of an ancient and venerable sociological principle, which is that what people believe is likely to be true in its consequences (Thomas and Znaniecki 1920). In the context of social protection, though, it is only a half truth. If people believe that eating beef is going to give them CJD, they are going to avoid eating beef, and they are going to demand some kind of protection. That changes the pattern of behaviour, and it has implications for policy, though – despite the sociological nostrum – the belief does not make the probability of getting CJD from beef any higher; indeed, it should be expected to reduce the number of cases of harm caused by beef, including the thousands of cases of people who have to go into hospital because they have choked while eating the stuff (see Table 2.1). Conversely, if people are ignorant of risks, they do not become less at risk – they become more so. The things that people believe have consequences, but they do not have to be true.

The misconceptions people have about risk are important. If people started treating carpets, armchairs and trousers with the apprehension they deserve, life would be very difficult. We 'know' that lawnmowers and chip pans are dangerous, but there are far more accidents with televisions and vacuum cleaners. The risks run by people in everyday life are complex. Table 2.1 shows data from the Home Accident Surveillance System, which estimates the incidence of accidents of different kinds, both within and outside the home, on the basis of admissions to a selection of Accident and Emergency Units (DTI, 2000).

There are several instructive points to make from this. The national figures are concerned with social risks in aggregate, not with individual risks. The total risk is clearly affected by the numbers of people exposed: chain saws and bouncing castles are dangerous because the numbers of accidents are seriously disproportionate to the number of users; tea cosies, a very practical way of scalding unsuspecting tea addicts with shaky hands, only appear safe because no-one uses them any more. (Besides, comedian Jeremy Hardy comments, you have to remember that tea cosies are more frightened of you than you are of them.) Equally, some items may appear to be dangerous because they affect vulnerable people, such as old people who may have falls even on level ground: this is probably why carpets and baths have such a bad record. Some items appear safe because the damage they do is not usually the sort which leads to accidents (like computers and personal stereos). But there are also some evidently dangerous items, like bicycles (the figure in the table excludes road traffic accidents), trainers and car doors, and we continue to use them anyway.

Demands for a response to risk are usually formulated in terms of the risk to the individual, rather than the aggregate risk. If rat poison is thought of as more risky than a computer, it is true both because the seriousness of the risk is greater, and the marginal risk is higher. The marginal risk is probably the more important of the two; it matters not only what the overall risk is, but what the risk is of doing the thing next time. People dress much more frequently than they use a lawnmower, and the risks have to be adjusted accordingly. Related to this is the perceived degree of control over that risk; people who use chip pans generally are making a decision

Table 2.1 Factors associated with accidents leading to hospital admissions

Accidents involving	Number	National estimate
Bicycles	9348	182566
Carpets	9327	179410
Trainers (footwear)	6500	126945
Alcoholic drink	5338	104251
Car doors	2364	46169
Baths	1551	30291
Armchairs	957	18690
Meat	694	13554
Vegetables	633	12363
Televisions	536	10468
Vacuum cleaners	509	9941
Socks and tights	504	9843
Bouncing castles	400	7812
Lawnmowers	341	6659
Trousers	263	5137
Chip pans	228	4453
Cots	185	3613
Microwave ovens	94	1836
Tree trunks	91	1777
Computers	83	1621
Chain saws	66	1289
Sponges and loofahs	51	996
Rat poison	23	450
Gravestones	17	332
Paperclips	12	234
Personal stereos	7	137
Tea cosies	1	20

Source: selected from DTI (2000).

based on their perception of their ability to use one despite the well-known risk, and for the most part they seem to be right.

The main response to marginal risk is the reduction of risk, through preventative action. Some risks should not have to be borne, and many areas – most obviously food, fuel, housing, transport and public health – have been the subject of legislation intended to reduce the level of risk endured in everyday life. It also means that where a risk is perceived, there may be the option of stopping it from occurring, often by banning the activity which brings it about. I started writing this piece after listening to a radio report arguing for banning baby walkers, which cause an estimated 3700 accidents a year.

There is, though, another calculation to consider: the balance of risks and benefits. People use cars, despite the risks, because personal transport is vital to do other things. The estimated 265,000 people admitted to hospital after falling down stairs has not led to a general demand to close down staircases, or even to redesign them. Where the perceived benefit is high, or the cost of avoidance is too great, the central issue for social policy is not risk avoidance, but risk management – a reduction not in the possibility of events occurring, but in the potential consequences.

One of the principal means of protecting people against harmful consequences is the pooling of risk – either through insurance or through collective social provision. The pooling of risk has some important limitations. The problems of 'adverse selection' and 'moral hazard' apply uniquely to issues of risk – not to the other forms of insecurity being considered in this chapter. Adverse selection occurs because some people are more at risk than others, and it may be in the interests of others to exclude people at high risk – for example, refusing health care to older people. This is identified with 'cream-skimming' in private insurance, but the same principle applies throughout the public sector; in conditions of scarcity, it may be necessary to ration, and rationing commonly requires choices between more serious and demanding cases and cases with lower levels of need. Moral hazard is used principally to refer to cases in which individuals voluntarily subject themselves to risk, which vitiates the contract with others in a solidaristic community: people who participate in extreme sports, for example, may not be considered to justify pooled risks on equal terms with others. (Moral hazard is also importantly 'moral', because a range of actions – including drug addiction, suicide and criminal violence – offend moral codes; moral obligations are liable to be suspended when other moral rules are breached. This can apply to other forms of social protection besides those which depend on pooled risk.)

Although insurance is the paradigmatic form of social protection against contingencies, it is not the only option. Alternatives include universal services, such as the NHS; minimum guarantees, such as Income Support in the UK; and even discretionary systems (like community care or *Aide Sociale* in France). The common principle is generally described in terms of 'solidarity', but the concept of solidarity is imprecise, and might also refer to redistribution.

Vulnerability

Vulnerability is closely related to risk, though there are important distinctions between them. People are at risk if something negative might happen. People are vulnerable when, if something negative happens, it will damage them; vulnerability is defined by the damage, not the risk. People who are at risk are often vulnerable, but not always; many more people are vulnerable than those who are at risk. A person who is in a high-paid, low-security occupation (like executive management) is at risk, but not vulnerable; a person who is in secure, low-paid employment (like, say, a local authority clerk), but is not covered for housing costs in the event of unemployment, is vulnerable but not at risk. This is important for social policy, because it is vulnerability, not risk, which is the principal subject of social protection. This is almost a tautology, because vulnerability can be seen as the absence of protection; vulnerability and protection are opposites. The identification of vulnerability with a need for protection has, however, a practical implication: people who are at risk but not vulnerable are not usually the subject of social protection measures. State and mutualist systems do not generally protect people against risks like business failure, bad debt, or loss of property value. (There are many exceptions, because there are circumstances where such risks make people vulnerable, and support for agriculture or ex-soldiers are often presented as forms of social protection.)

Poor people are, notoriously, more vulnerable than many others. But vulnerability is not equivalent to poverty, and it is possible to construct circumstances in which richer people are more vulnerable than poor ones. This is particularly important in developing countries, where the effect of increasing resources is also to increase vulnerability.

> Diversified subsistence farmers may be poor but are not vulnerable. When they enter the market by selling specialised cash crops, or raising their earnings by incurring debts, or investing in risky ventures, their incomes rise, but they become vulnerable. There are trade-offs between poverty and vulnerability (or between security and income).
>
> (Streeten 1995)

A parallel process is visible in developed countries, where the high level of specialization has made certain groups of workers – such as workers in heavy industry, for instance miners, steel workers or shipbuilders – especially vulnerable to changes in the structure of the economy. People's circumstances become more robust when they have a wider range of options; industrial training and re-deployment schemes are supposed to reduce vulnerability. The Social Fund of the European Union, which is geared to the protection of people in displaced industries, exists largely to provide support of this kind.

Vulnerability implies, simply enough, a lack of shielding against negative consequences, and the response to vulnerability is principally to offer this kind of shielding. People generally look for one of three kinds of arrangement. The first is restitution: people want to have the negative consequences nullified or dealt with. People who break a leg generally want to have their leg fixed. Often this implies the provision of a service, rather than a financial payment, though in many cases finance is a viable way of meeting the need – for example, protecting someone against losing a house by paying the mortgage. Funeral insurance is a way of dealing with problems (death can hardly be nullified); prior payment and coverage ensures a smooth, relatively painless process for the bereaved.

The second arrangement is to be compensated. Compensation usually involves a financial payment offered as a substitute for whatever is lost. (I say 'usually' because there are other forms of compensation – like an artificial limb for an amputee.) Compensation is generally an inferior option to restitution; even if the compensation is generous, the negative consequences are still suffered.

The third option is to be maintained. In France, health insurance generally covers most of the cost of health care, and makes some daily allowance for sickness, but there is still a shortfall. People join mutual insurance societies (the *mutualités*) to make up the difference – not just the out of pocket cost, but the remainder of income foregone which is not covered by health insurance. This is a voluntary supplement, but most of the people in France are covered.

States of dependency

The kinds of risk which insurance protects against are often unpredictable, and they affect a minority of people. But insurance-type arrangements are also made for conditions which can hardly be described in the same language: examples are funeral insurance (everyone dies) and pensions (because most people live to claim). These 'states of dependency' – the term is Titmuss's – are largely predictable, and (as Titmuss noted) fundamental to welfare provision (Titmuss 1963: 42).

In principle, there are important differences between protection against risk and provision for states of dependency. The coverage of risk works by pooling risks and resources, and allocating benefits from the pool. It follows that the primary purpose of protection against contingencies is redistributive. By contrast, in circumstances where the coverage of conditions of dependency is based on the same method, the allocated benefits have more or less to equal the contributions. This means that the principle ceases to be risk pooling, and becomes one of income smoothing – saving at one point in order to benefit at another. It is complicated by two other principles – solidaristic redistribution, where this occurs, and 'loading', which refers to added costs for operation, management and profit. These are both factors which may (unlike coverage for risk) lead people to prefer individual coverage (Culyer 1991). There are some associated elements of risk, especially uncertainty about the length of dependency. There is also commonly some potential for redistribution even in strictly funded, individualistic pension schemes, because some people will die and others will be unable to claim. The mechanisms of support which prepare for them are often the same as those which protect people against contingencies. For example, either scheme could work by dynamization – using resources from contributors now in order to pay for current beneficiaries, while relying on future contributors to meet future commitments.

Because of the differences in principle, there are also differences in practice. In the UK, the post-war welfare state attempted to provide for both forms of insecurity through contingent general rights – that is, rights available to all people in defined contingencies. Beveridgean systems have provided universal coverage at a low level, which has worked relatively well for some groups – notably in health care – but badly for others, notably pensions. In Bismarckian schemes, by contrast, insecurity is dealt with for preference through individualized, particular rights – that is, rights which are specific to the contributing individual. Social protection in much of continental Europe has provided relatively generous pensions but has notable gaps in coverage for the poorest (which is the rationale for the extension of measures for social inclusion). This implies a case for particular rights for pensioners and general rights for other contingencies such as health, and this pattern is being adopted by a number of countries, including the UK itself and the southern

European states. (The particularist aspects of southern Europe are well known (Ferrera 1996), but Italy, Spain and Portugal have also moved towards universal health provision.)

Precariousness

Finally, there is a special form of vulnerability which is related to the economic market. This is the situation which in France is referred to as '*précarité*' (e.g. in Milano 1992). (I have translated this, awkwardly, as 'precariousness'; 'instability' may be a better translation, but the term in English has a moral overtone which is probably best avoided.) Precariousness occurs in a range of different social contexts and labour markets, and different adaptations to circumstances may be expected from those who are sub-employed as well as different policy responses to the problems. The idea of 'dual' labour markets rests on a distinction between the type and character of labour undertaken by people in different parts of the economy, and points to the consistent disadvantages suffered by certain categories of worker. In the USA, a further distinction has been made between those who are employed, in any part of the market, and those who are sub-employed (Matza and Miller 1976). The concept of sub-employment refers to people who have a marginal position in the labour market. Marginal groups include migrant workers, single parents, some disabled people, and many people with low employment status or skills, who may find themselves employed only casually, intermittently or for limited periods of time. Their work is of low status and earning power; when work is scarce, they are likely to be unemployed. As a result, they are likely to move through various types of ephemeral labour, including temporary employment, casual labour and work in which they are unable to maintain any tenure, as well as experiencing periodic spells of unemployment. (There is some similarity between this and the 'individualized' circumstances which Beck is referring to, but this is a structural aspect of labour markets, applying only to certain sections of the population.)

This discussion has sometimes been related to the concept of an 'underclass'. Gallie suggests that the central weakness of underclass theory is that few groups seem to possess the level of stability implied by the representation of the underclass (Gallie 1998: 473–4). The ephemeral nature of their situations, and the complexity of changing patterns of employment, has made it difficult to identify patterns of sub-employment clearly in empirical terms. However, work by Morris and Irwin identifies a distinct set of patterns of marginal employment (Morris and Irwin 1992). Morris has discussed this work primarily in the framework of a critique of underclass theory (Morris 1994), but the identification of these patterns is important in its own right. If class is understood in economic terms, it is precisely the structured instability of their circumstances which defines people as members of a different class.

Social protection systems nowadays rarely address the issue of economic marginality. The Beveridge scheme in the UK was developed with intermittent and casual work very much in mind, and initially the rules for National Insurance cover, including daily payment of benefit and linking rules between periods of repeated short-term unemployment, were intended to cover the situation. (In the past, the cases were referred to as RSTCs, or Repeated Short-Term Claimants; but the last time I discussed the issue with the local Benefits Agency, they had stopped keeping these files distinctly.) The administrative problems of this kind of intensive case management, coupled with the relative growth of long-term unemployment, have made this kind of response seem increasingly less appropriate, and benefit rules have gradually been modified to allow for aggregation of resources and the establishment of earnings limits by the week. In France, resources and work are aggregated over much longer periods (one month for benefits, three months for contributions), which greatly reduces administration but at the same time can lead to substantial delays in responsiveness.

Current systems of social protection are not geared to cope with unstable circumstances, and they are liable to aggravate the problems of sub-employment. People who work intermittently are subject not only to increased administration, but are liable to penalization for leaving employment, delays in benefit delivery, and suspicion of fraud. There is a recurrent problem with overpayment of housing benefit (because people may be entitled at some times and not at others), and, where there are minimum waiting periods (such as the period necessary for owner-occupiers to qualify for mortgage interest payments) benefits may be lost.

Conclusion: responding to insecurity

The kinds of insecurity which people are protecting against are complex, and it is not possible to reduce them to a simple formula. There is a tendency to reduce many of these complexities to financial benefits, because that is the way that many social protection systems respond to the problems, but clearly the range of activities which might be affected is wide. A broad term like 'health' can cover a wide range of physical conditions, emotional distress and needs for social care. People who retire in old age commonly look for a pension, but a pension alone is unlikely to be sufficient to provide security; other issues which need to be considered are health care, social care and issues related to death and succession.

The issues raised by insecurity go well beyond issues of income and wealth. They include the protection of personal independence, both physical and material; the protection of a person's lifestyle, through measures to protect property, to provide domestic help or to allow for long-term residential care; and the protection of the interests of dependants and successors. It is unwise to assume that these concerns are of lesser importance than other forms of risk; it is not at all clear, for example, that old people value their own health above the property interests of their successors.

Social policies are not necessarily likely to respond to claims based on insecurity. In relation to the extension of social protection, the story is mixed. There are examples of developing provision: the most notable cases are the growth of coverage of medical care, which in most countries in Europe has become virtually universal, and the increasing emphasis on social inclusion, which has led to the extension of coverage in France, Italy, Portugal and northern Spain. Protection in the labour market, protection for states of dependency and minimum income guarantees are widespread. But, in the name of the market, there are also strong examples of a retreat from other measures – the attempt to reduce risk through public health, or to reduce lack of basic security through the provision of housing. There has been a tendency, in attempts to retrench the welfare state, to reduce the scope of social protection, emphasizing greater need rather than insecurity. Part of this trend has been a reduction in universal forms of income maintenance in favour of residual ones (Andries 1996).

In terms of the forms of insecurity considered in the first part of this chapter, the shift to residualism relates most strongly to two forms. One is protection against a lack of basic security, which could be done universally or selectively. The other is protection against states of dependency – important in provision for old age, family policy and disability. In relation to risk, the arguments are mixed, but the extension of health coverage suggests a countervailing trend. In relation to the other forms of insecurity – vulnerability and precariousness – the response of social protection systems has always been restricted, and the discovery that such restrictions largely continue to apply should be unsurprising.

Probably the main lesson for social policy to draw from this analysis is that one method does not fit every case. Measures which are appropriate for risk do not necessarily provide basic security; measures which provide basic security do not necessarily protect people who are vulnerable; measures for people who are vulnerable do not necessarily cover people in precarious situations. In most cases, provision of one kind will generally help the others to some degree; even limited protection against vulnerability helps to protect against basic insecurity to some degree (which is the central argument for universal benefits). Protection against basic insecurity helps every other sort of insecurity: the stronger the foundation, the better the protection. In the special case of precariousness, however, measures which improve the security of some may make the problems worse for others; this happens because many measures designed to protect against risk, including minimum income guarantees and social insurance, rely on a clear definition of circumstances which may not be possible.

References

Andries, M. (1996) 'The politics of targeting: the Belgian case', *Journal of European Social Policy* 6(3): 209–23.

Baldwin, P. (1990) *The politics of social solidarity*, Cambridge: Cambridge University Press.

Beck, U. (1992) *Risk Society*, London: Sage.

—— (1997) *Reinventing politics*, Oxford: Polity Press.

Culyer, A. (1991) 'The normative economics of health care: finance and provision', in

A. McGuire, P. Fenn and K. Mayhew (eds), *Providing health care*, Oxford: Oxford University Press.

DTI, Department of Trade and Industry (2000) *Home Accident Survey System including leisure activities: 22nd Annual Report 1998 data*, London: DTI.

Duffy, K. (1995) Social exclusion and human dignity in Europe, Strasbourg: Council of Europe CDPS(95) 1 Rev.

Drèze, J. and Sen, A. (1989) *Hunger and public action*, Oxford: Clarendon Press.

Ferrera, M. (1996) 'The "Southern Model" of welfare in social Europe', *Journal of European Social Policy* 6(1): 17–37.

Gallie, D. (1998) *Employment in Britain*, Oxford: Blackwell.

Giddens, A. (1994) *Beyond left and right*, Cambridge: Polity Press.

Leach, E. (ed.) (1960) *Aspects of caste in South India, Ceylon and North-west Pakistan*, Cambridge: Cambridge University Press.

Matza, D. and Miller, H. (1976) 'Poverty and proletariat', in R. Merton and R. Nisbet (eds) *Contemporary social problems*, New York: Harcourt Brace Jovanovich, 4th edition.

Milano, S. (1992) *La pauvreté dans les pays riches*, Paris: Nathan.

Morris, L. and Irwin, S. (1992) 'Employment histories and the concept of the underclass', *Sociology* 26(3): 401–20.

—— (1994) *Dangerous classes*, London: Routledge.

Mullard, M. and Spicker, P. (1998) *Social policy in a changing society*, London: Routledge.

Steuer, M. (1998) 'A little too risky', *LSE Magazine* 10(1): 15–16.

Streeten, P. (1995) Comments on 'The framework of ILO action against poverty', in G. Rodgers (ed.), *The poverty agenda and the ILO*, Geneva: International Labour Office.

Thomas, W. and Znaniecki, F. (1920) *The Polish peasant in Europe and America*, Chicago: Chicago University Press.

Titmuss, R. (1963) 'The Social Division of Welfare', in *Essays on the Welfare State*, London: Unwin.

Chapter 3

Transparent and messy contracts – how do they serve social security?

Zsuzsa Ferge[1]

> Apparent inconsistencies are a source of stability, achieved through a compromise which is not dictated by logic.
>
> (Marshall 1965:134)

Introduction and overview

Background to the argument

Modern welfare states have produced institutions that can serve several social objectives by reconciling divergent interests (Baldwin 1990). The social contracts[2] forged in the last 150 years offer protection against many risks of the market, and many uncertainties of human life. These contracts usually refer to new or renewed political agreements between the government and citizens on broad social issues. The commitments enshrined in these contracts are not necessarily legally enforceable, yet they shape the behaviour of both sides. They also serve social integration and social justice. Social insurance schemes and labour rights belong to these institutions. The political processes shaping them use civil and political rights to acquire and to strengthen social and economic rights. The development of welfare institutions is thereby intricately related to the advancement of social citizenship.

The trends of globalization and the dominant ideology driving them are inimical to social contracts. Economic arguments stress that such contracts are unsustainable under the conditions of global competition. They affirm that the liberated market will produce growth automatically trickling down and benefiting the poor (Dollard and Kraay 2000). A more sophisticated version of the economic approach (apparently concerned with poverty reduction) advocates a

> new broad definition of Social Protection, SP, (that) centers on the concept of social risk management (SRM). *SP consists of public interventions (i) to assist individual households and communities better manage risk, and (ii) to provide support to the critically poor.*
>
> (Holzmann and Jorgensen 2000: 9, emphasis in the original)

The role of public intervention is thereby reduced to creating a legal framework for the management of risk. This will – among other things – offer the poor opportunities to engage in high risk/high return activities. The other public function is to help the 'critically poor', that is those 'who could not provide for themselves even if employment opportunities did exist'.

(Holzmann and Jorgensen 2000:10)

Economic arguments about the unsustainability of social contracts are completed by political ones invoking political sustainability. It is suggested that individual savings accounts 'may be more resilient to political risk' than 'unfunded and publicly managed provisions' for unemployment or health (Holzmann and Jorgensen 2000: 23).

This chapter is prompted by yet another criticism directed against social insurance schemes that claim that these schemes are unclear and therefore unstable:

> The design of every pension system . . . has a built-in conflict of objectives. Ideally one would want to enable everyone to reconstitute a target share of their own career earnings in retirement. At the same time, civilised societies want some floor to be placed below everyone's living standard in retirement, regardless of what they actually earned and contributed. Any attempt to achieve both objectives – intertemporal insurance and interpersonal distribution – in a single 'pension pillar' involves *messy and dynamically unstable compromises*.
>
> (World Bank 1995: 31, my emphasis)

Compromises that attempt to reconcile conflicting interests are indeed necessarily unstable. In order to gain permanence and legitimization their terms have constantly to be readjusted to the changing field of forces and to altering conditions. Without democratically negotiated compromises the stronger interests will prevail with possibly fatal consequences. Apparently messy contracts are currently under this threat.

The main objective of this chapter is thus to take a closer look at the alleged messiness of social contracts by deconstructing and reconstructing the concept.

The structure of the chapter

The messiness of social contracts is real enough. I think though that this is not their weakness but their strength. They combine different principles of access to resources or allocative principles.[3] All of them are accepted as legitimate organizers of social life. Their mixing allows compromises between various values and interests.

Four basic allocative principles are distinguished and described in some detail on pp. 34–6. All of them generate 'single-principle' patterns of transactions. The allocative principles are altruism or charity, reciprocity, the market principle, and citizens' rights. These categories intentionally remind one of Karl Polanyi's patterns of integration. Later in the chapter I make extensive use of his insights on a 'pure' market (Polanyi 1944). However, I try to make a conceptual distinction between the patterns of transactions and the principles informing them. This allows me to separate the single principles and the complex patterns. This approach means that I put Polanyi's three basic concepts of reciprocity, redistribution and the market in a different context. Charity underpins one-sided giving or almsgiving; reciprocity implies the donation of service or gift and normatively expected counter-service; the market principle is prevalent on a self-regulating, 'pure' market; and citizens' rights in the sense put forward by Marshall (1965) is the foundation of some universal (public) benefits. The transactions based on the three last principles take the form of contracts, including written contracts and ethically binding promises.

Some characteristics of the single principle patterns are briefly described on pp. 36–9, namely the type of the power relations operating in them; the economic or non-economic rationality orienting them; their impact on social integration; their potential coverage; and the adequacy of the need satisfaction they provide.

In real life the allocative principles may operate singly, or they may be combined. The next section argues that single principle transactions were not well adapted to the conditions of modern complex societies. Combinations have been worked out to enhance their social effectiveness. When reciprocity was combined for instance with rights and/or the market principle as in the labour contract or in social insurance, the allocative pattern improved. Meanwhile the contract has become 'messy'. These messy contracts can accommodate diverse, often conflicting purposes and interests, eventually also in the interest of the weaker partners.

The neo-liberal approach is discrediting the present multi-principle and multi-purpose institutions of social protection. Alternatives described on pp. 42–4 offer to replace the messy contracts by traditional single-principle patterns like pure charity (the safety net) or by pure market solutions. Some new messy contracts are also on offer in which citizens and their rights are overshadowed by an authoritarian power.

The final section summarizes the argument put forward in this chapter. It leaves open the question of whether the old messy contracts may be recast, or whether other acceptable alternatives may be found.

Description of the single allocative principles

There are individual entitlements to resources – achievement, merit, inheritance, luck – that are widely recognized as important. The collective or societal legitimating allocative principles are less often discussed. I emphasize legitimacy because this chapter focuses on socially accepted ways of need satisfaction. Legitimacy means that the principle is in accordance with the law (unlike theft) and it is accepted as normal practice by the huge majority of citizens (unlike gambling).

Altruism

Altruism, the 'selfless' love of others, is a widely accepted ethical legitimating principle of charitable almsgiving. In modern times, charitable giving as a micro-level transaction has been institutionalized on the macro-level as social assistance.

Charitable giving – whether private alms giving or public assistance – is by definition one-sided giving. It assumes a substantively asymmetrical relationship, and the act itself reinforces the inequality. The one-sided giving may make a moral debtor of the receiver who, at the least, owes humble gratitude to the generous benefactor. In the 'economics of charitable giving', in earlier times the main reward was, of course, salvation (Castel 1995: 47). In modern times an important symbolic gain is the sense of social superiority, social prestige attached to philanthropy, and/or moral self-righteousness.

The losses for the beneficiaries are also significant. The loss of self-esteem and of any claim for social recognition may be the most important. In the early schemes, the loss of political rights by the poor was a self-evident corollary of assistance. The curtailment of rights is less explicit in our days. Nevertheless, the asymmetry built into assistance schemes undermines equal citizenship. Even if law defines eligibility, the claimant remains a petitioner:[4] s/he has to ask for rights that are granted self-evidently for others. The inequality built into social assistance is not in line with the diminishing hierarchies seen as a corollary of modernity and post-modernity either. The constantly reaffirmed social inferiority of the beneficiary generates a vicious spiral. It may well be that the so-called dependency culture is an end product of this spiral, the result of the continuous loss of face *vis-à-vis* others, and of the loss of faith in oneself.

Allegations about the moral harms of assistance always threatened the legitimacy of the scheme. Social assistance was always jeopardized by the problem of the able-bodied poor. When their number grew, altruism reached its limits. Various rationales and instruments were invented to ease the load on the assistance rolls.

Reciprocity

Reciprocity is the legitimating principle of transactions (donation and expected counter-donation) that have the following characteristics: they take place outside the market; the partners are seen as social equals; the equivalence of the goods or services exchanged is not exactly calculated; there is a time gap between giving and taking; and economic profit is excluded from the transaction.

In the case of reciprocity (as Polanyi (1944) suggests) the transaction itself is constructed in such a way as to assure or produce symmetry in a substantive sense. The social, ethical or even affective contents that strengthen social bonds are organic features of the transaction. Reciprocity has long ceased to be a dominant pattern of integration, but it still flourishes within the extended family; it also survives in friendly societies, in gift relations, or in the mutual exchange of services.

A reciprocal relationship does not guarantee the exchange of equal values: the objects of the exchange may not even be precisely commensurable. There is no written contract with precise terms but a deep-rooted sense of mutual obligation. Mutual trust that the obligation will be honoured is essential when there is no written contract and there is a time gap between giving and taking. Trust is also nurtured by the shared feeling of fairness, excluding a one-sided substantial economic (or other) gain. Reciprocity continues to mean, up to the present, that the economic kernel is enmeshed in social bonds.

All these characteristics apply to the 'spontaneous solidarity' emerging in small communities, implying face-to-face relationships. When societies become large and dense, with long chains of interdependencies that are increasingly impersonal (de Swaan 1988), reciprocity reappears in a new guise. Some of its essential features may survive as 'macro-level solidarity', in the form of unwritten societal contracts; the contract between generations built into publicly managed redistributive schemes is one example.

The market

The market was originally no more than the place of barter or of the occasional buying and selling of goods. With the advent of the market society it has become an institution shaping the whole organization of society. This creates a new situation: 'Instead of the economy being embedded in social relations, social relations are embedded in the economic system' (Polanyi 1944: 57).

The market principle informs transactions that are shaped in economic terms by supply and demand, with prices ultimately defined by the opportunity costs of the partners. In sociological terms, it is economic activity based on freedom of property, of labour and of contract, geared by unlimited 'free' competition, and aiming at profit maximization.

A market contract is usually described as a relationship between free and equal partners, a symmetrical relationship *par excellence*. The symmetry certainly prevails in a legal sense. Yet the bargaining position of the partners impacts on the terms and the outcome of the contract. This position depends on the equilibrium/ disequilibrium of supply and demand; on how well the contracting partners are organized (in monopolies, in trade unions, and so on); on each partner's relationship to the central power; on the urgency of the need of one of the partners that may undermine his/her ability to drive a hard bargain. This last problem is translated in neutral economic terms as the opportunity cost paid by one of the partners. In social terms it means that the formally equal market relations may be highly asymmetrical in a substantive sense.

Citizens' rights

Citizens' rights include civil, political and social rights. In Marshall's terms, social rights give access to 'the whole range from the right to a modicum of economic welfare and security to the right to share to the full in the social heritage and to live the life of a civilised being according to the standards prevailing in society' (Marshall 1965: 78). Social citizenship assures dignity because rights remove the stigma from help.

Citizens' rights form the allocative principle of all universal benefits, including in their ideal typical variant of a universal allocation to which all citizens are entitled. The idea of a basic income for all may be traced back to a number of egalitarian thinkers from Tom Paine (1737–1809) through Charles Fourier, an early socialist (1772–1837), to Lady Rhys-Williams writing in the 1940s (Rhys-Williams 1942). Its current concept seems to owe more to Marshall's approach to social citizenship than to earlier formulations. Marshall made a clear distinction between the early 'social rights' embodied for instance in the Poor Laws and modern social rights that are part of a complex of citizenship rights. His argument suggests that social rights may predate citizenship rights. However, they may crumble very easily if secure civil and political rights do not back them (Marshall 1965: 86–9).[5]

The universal allocation or basic income scheme is currently on the agenda as an alternative to all other forms of social provisions. Over the last few decades, it has been conceptualized as an allocative principle based squarely and singly on citizens' rights, as a truly unconditional transfer to every member of society (van Parijs 1995).

Some characteristics of the single-principle transactions

Power relations

The power relations shaping the various single-principle transactions described above differ profoundly. Here only a simplified overview is offered:

- In the case of altruism there is always a hierarchical, asymmetrical relationship between the giver and the taker.
- Reciprocity by definition is based on, and creates, symmetrical relationships. This does not imply that there are no unequal power positions in society at large. Nevertheless the reciprocal transaction has to take place between those who occupy a similar position within the hierarchy.
- The power relations within a market contract are meant to be formally symmetrical, but they may remain substantively very unequal.
- The social acceptance of citizens' rights assumes the existence of a modern state with necessarily unequal power relations. However citizens' rights, and among them social rights, may be stronger or weaker depending on the protective power of democratic arrangements, on the strength of civil and political rights; on the strength of ideologies for and against positive rights; and of course on what the constituency holds about their legitimacy.

A simplified picture of the power inequalities related to the different single allocative principles is given in Figure 3.1.

Principles	The power relationship is		The symmetry is	
	symmetrical	asymmetrical	only formal	also substantive
Altruism		*		
Reciprocity	*			*
Self-regulating market	*		*	
Citizens' rights	*		* (?)	*(?)

Figure 3.1 Symmetry–asymmetry of power relationships related to allocative principles

* The asterisks indicate only the presence of a given characteristic without hinting as to its prevalence.

(?) A question mark indicates indetermination: whether symmetry is only formal or also substantive depends on the broader social context.

Economic and other rationalities

All of the transactions described above have an economic kernel: they all assure access to goods. The rationality operating within the transaction, however, may not be exclusively the formal economic rationality aiming at profit optimization.

- Altruism may be imbued with moral obligation or human sensitivity, it may aim at some transcendent reward, or may be motivated simply by fear of social unrest. In this sense there is an underlying economic rationality: it may be cheaper to pre-empt or prevent social unrest than to curb it afterwards. This rationality is external to the transaction, though.
- In the case of reciprocity, the substantive economic rationality may be openly acknowledged. It may however serve its original purpose, social cohesion, only if it completely foregoes formal economic rationality.
- By definition, the unfettered market is moved by formal economic rationality.
- Citizens' rights cannot be argued for on grounds of economic rationality: they are rooted in political, ethical and social considerations. Economic rationality may play an important role but again as an external condition, for instance in the form of affordability.

An imaginary scale may be constructed. Market rationality or the market principle may be placed at one end of the scale, with non-contractual, one-sided almsgiving at the other extreme. Somewhere in the middle of the scale a delicate balance may exist between economic and ethical or social (value) rationalities: reciprocity may be an example. The relationship between the different rationalities and the allocative principles is sketched in Figure 3.2. This figure also shows the assumed impact of the allocative principles on system integration and on social integration (Lockwood 1964).

	The dominant rationality – the two extremes		The supposed impact	
	economic	moral, social, sometimes affective	on system integration	on social integration
Altruism		*		*
Reciprocity	*	*	*	*
Self-regulating market	*		*	
Citizens' rights		*	*	*

Figure 3.2 Rationality and integrative role related to allocative principles

* The asterisks indicate only the presence of a given characteristic without hinting as to its prevalence.

Coverage and adequacy

Social citizenship requires public schemes with complete or almost complete coverage of citizens that meet a socially acceptable level of need satisfaction. The adequacy of standards (Veit-Wilson 1998) refers to how well needs are covered. Single-principle transactions may not serve well coverage and adequacy.

- Charity has low potential for covering the majority. It assumes face-to-face contacts, or at least short chains of interdependence. Nobody can assure or guarantee that such contacts will spread over the whole community. Indeed, they have to be voluntary transactions: law cannot enforce them. Social assistance may reach, at least in theory, all the 'needy', albeit in practice this is almost impossible. As for adequacy, in the case of charity the giver decides the size of the donation in an arbitrary way that may or may not be commensurate with the needs of the recipient. Uncertainty is part of this deal. The standards of assistance are seldom adequate: the less eligibility principle looms large in most modern societies.
- The potential coverage of reciprocity is similar to that of charity. The outcome of reciprocity is indeterminate, from the perspective of adequacy, and security is built into the deal.

- In principle, the self-regulating market reaches everybody. In practice many may be excluded. The best known form of the exclusion from the market is of course poverty, the inability to pay for needs seen as essential for social citizenship. Labour market imbalances form a major cause of the inability to acquire resources and hence of the inability to pay. Adequacy or the need of the partners is not a valid consideration in pure market contracts and uncertainty is endemic. Other causes of exclusion may be personal, political, or even spatial (Atkinson 1998).
- Access through citizens' rights is designed to cover everybody. The level of adequacy and the stability of benefits assured by citizens' rights may depend on the availability of economic resources, but they are essentially political matters.

Thus, all the single-principle patterns have weaknesses. They create or strengthen substantive inequality (charity and the market); their coverage may be restricted (charity and reciprocity); their social legitimization may be defective (the market and citizens' rights); their practical adequacy is always questionable; and the security they offer is usually limited or shaky.

Messy contracts

The shortcomings of single allocative principles explain the emergence of more complex patterns intertwining several of the above principles. The most important new constructs are the modern labour contract and social insurance. In both cases the pure market principle is 'messed with'. The harshness of the market is moderated through reciprocity (or solidarity) and social rights. Coverage may improve because of the enforceability of the schemes. Adequacy is served by the broader coverage itself, as strong interests also become included. The new collective structures empower the weaker partners and reduce the risk of direct economic or political influence on the schemes. Current attacks on social insurance often invoke the dangers of arbitrary political (state) intervention. They invariably fail to mention, though, the stabilizing potential of hard-won legitimacy, and the political protection represented by pluralistic and relatively independent governing bodies. Examples of the allocative principles of single or multi-principle patterns are given in Figure 3.3.

Labour contracts

The formally and legally equal contracting partners of the market may sign economic contracts entailing disproportionate advantages for one of them. This applies particularly strongly to the labour market. As long as the unequal partners face each other without some non-market support for the weaker partner, labour remains a pure commodity that is sold cheaply or not sold at all.

Contract-law cannot solve the riddle of the discrepancy between the formal symmetry and the substantive asymmetry. It recognizes some instances of unfairly

Examples of patterns of transactions	Legitimating principle			
	Altruism	Reciprocity or solidarity	Self-regulating market	Citizens' rights
Traditional charitable donation	*			
Gifts; help within the community	*	*		
'Pure' market exchange			*	
Modern social assistance	*			*
Labour contract		*	*	*
Social insurance	*	*	*	*
Basic income				*
Participation income		*		*

Figure 3.3 The legitimating allocative principles in the case of different real-life transactions

one-sided agreements as in tort, duress, or unconsciability (Fried 1981: 5). However, contractual law treats these events as random, individual cases – not as a structurally determined, socially recurrent situation. In the real labour market though, the unequal position of the partners is not the exception but the rule.

Hence the Weberian distinction between formal law and substantive law or substantive justice is important. Formal law assures calculability and unambiguity, and guarantees the application of rules 'without regard for persons' (Gerth and Mills 1946: 215). This 'inhumanity' may clash with sentiments, ethical considerations or popular feelings about justice:

> The propertyless masses especially are not served by a formal 'equality before the law' and a 'calculable' adjudication and administration as demanded by the 'bourgeois' interests. Naturally, in their eyes, justice and administration should serve to compensate for their economic and social life-opportunities in the face of the propertied classes. Justice and administration can fulfil this

function only if they assume an informal character to a far-reaching extent. It must be informal because it is substantively 'ethical' ('Kadi-justice').

(Gerth and Mills 1946: 221)

Social law, and in particular labour law, succeeded in translating many informal ethical considerations into calculable legal dispositions. In other words 'Kadi-justice' has to some extent been formalized. Thus social and labour law could be adapted to the requirements of the market, but they have changed to some degree the logic of the market itself.

Since the end of the nineteenth century, and in particular since 1945, individual labour contracts, previously characterized by the defencelessness of workers, have been increasingly surrounded by collective, protective rules. According to Supiot (1995), all work accomplished in the labour market should be linked to rights and duties towards the collectivity within a solidaristic system. The collective structures created by protective legislation indeed transformed the scene. They empower labour to some extent and reduce the power inequality between the 'social partners'. They also confer an acceptable social status and dignity to labour (Castel 1995).

With protective legislation the pure labour contract certainly becomes messy. The supply and demand equilibrium is distorted, usually in favour of labour. The interests that thereby are harmed understandably attack the protective role of legal arrangements. The alleged reasons are economic, such as sustainability or competitiveness. The proposed instrument is deregulation or rather, as Standing (1999) explains, re-regulation adjusted to the changing power constellation.

The case of pension insurance

Public pension insurance is a blatant example of a messy contract. On the face of it, a modern public pension scheme is simply an institution of equivalent transfers between the economically active and retired earners. It may be seen as inter-temporal redistribution in which actuarial correctness assures market conformity. Reality is less simple, though. The so-called equivalence principle may have been relatively pronounced in the early (funded) Bismarckian schemes. Later, and particularly after 1945 when most European countries switched to public pay-as-you-go schemes, departures from this principle have multiplied.

A public earnings-related pay-as-you-go scheme has, at present, not only economic, but (explicit or implicit) social, political and ethical objectives. It serves security in old age and it endeavours to assure adequacy of need coverage in old age. Gender equality was seriously harmed by the early schemes, but there are now efforts to promote it, such as through the European Union. The virtual or real collective capital represented by the funds serves the empowerment of the insured. Pension rights rooted in the wage relation transfer the status or identity of the worker to the pensioner and thereby may assure some dignity in old age.

In these schemes, the freedom of contract assured by formal law is harmed. The agents are no more formally free: joining is in most European (and some other) countries mandatory. The freedom for gaining profit is also harmed. In the case of a market insurance contract private profit seeking is a legitimate concern. In social insurance it is not.

The advantages of public pension schemes materialize mainly when the middle strata have become interested enough to accept the compulsion to join these schemes. Their inclusion improved standards. Economies of scale reduced the costs. Moreover the increased constituency strengthened public support and hence the legitimacy of the schemes. Meanwhile, interpersonal and intertemporal redistribution within the schemes has become fraught both with 'black lies' conducive to regressive redistribution, and 'white lies' producing positive redistribution in favour of the more disadvantaged groups.[6]

Accusations of 'messiness' in public pension insurance is, then, well founded. Yet I doubt that the combination of principles amounts to a sham or sophistry as suggested for instance by Hayek in connection with the social security program introduced in 1935 in the USA (Issing 1998: 15). They just take account of the complexity of human needs.

The dissolution and reinvention of messy contracts

I reviewed the arguments against public social security arrangements on p. 32. Such attacks are usually complemented by reform proposals. The best known recommendations are the curtailment of labour rights; the abandonment of the idea of the living wage;[7] stricter eligibility rules and lowering standards in public insurance; private 'money-purchase' schemes (named private pension schemes) for security in old age; private insurance or individual savings accounts for all other 'risks', more recently wrapped in terms of Social Risk Management; private charity; means-tested public assistance for those squeezed out from other schemes; and the termination of dispositions assuring rights without duties. In other words, mainly single-principle patterns are advocated, but only some of them. The neo-liberal agenda forcibly rejects citizens' rights as a single allocative principle.

In what follows I illustrate the discussion of changes in social contracts with the handling of unemployment. When and where unemployment has become high and lasting, the old messy contract of unemployment insurance has broken down.[8] Its underlying assumption about reciprocity could not be upheld any more. Then a search starts for functional alternatives.

In many countries the first move is to unload the beneficiaries from the overburdened scheme to some other institutionalized allocative pattern regarded as better fitted to accommodate masses. Disability or early retirement pension schemes seem adequate for this purpose. Eriksen and Palmer note for instance that in Sweden, 'Disability has been used as a means of exit from the labour market in response to actual or threatening unemployment' (Eriksen and Palmer 1997: 154). A similar solution was applied in the Netherlands and in many Central–Eastern European countries after the transition, Hungary among them.

The rapid increase in the number of pensioners overstrains solidarity: re-distribution within the scheme becomes too obvious. This kindles attacks on the messiness of the pattern.

A cleansing of the pension scheme may follow. The disability or age tests are made stricter. Those squeezed out from the insurance schemes may then get social assistance, swelling the assistance rolls. However, social assistance was not designed to receive masses either. Thus the vicious circle starts anew.

Meanwhile social assistance is the last resort. Its withdrawal means exclusion from all public help. This solution may not be acceptable for public norms (as is the case in Western Europe), or it may breed trouble (everywhere). Therefore a middle way has to be found between exclusion and the unconditional right to inclusion. At this point proposals emerge for new or very old messy solutions. Some of them attempt to pursue 'old' ideals of the welfare consensus such as symmetry, adequacy, inclusiveness, and dignity assured by rights. The French Revenu Minimum d'Insertion (minimum guaranteed income for social integration) may be seen as an experiment combining several allocative principles. It also links individualized 'treatment' to new, mainly local collective structures. This, however, is not only a rather costly solution. Empowerment is one of its explicit objectives, but the individualizing agenda works against it. Moreover, the goodwill motivating the scheme is hard to implement (Castel 1995: 418–34).

The cheaper alternative – and one that is spreading – is 'workfare', a new messy contract combining the market principle with alleged reciprocity or charity and legal coercion. This appears to be an authoritarian solution harming both security and freedom. Amartya Sen (2000: 2) recently wrote that 'global capitalist institutions show a distinct preference for orderly autocracies over the adversarial politics of democratic governance and the activist use of human rights'. This observation applies not only to global institutions but also to national ones, namely the nation-states increasingly influenced by global economic interests (Boyer and Drache 1996).

The workfare 'contract' may rightfully be termed a pseudo-reciprocal pseudo-contract. More often than not, this is not a real market contract: at least one of the agents is not freely entering the contract, so that even formal equality is harmed. It is not a regulated market contract either because it is not infused by labour rights and social rights. It is not reciprocity because it is not based on substantive equality. There is no time gap between giving and taking. Finally the ethical or trust element is absent. Goodin rightfully terms it immoral and hypocritical (Goodin 1998).

The demeaning, hypocritical and unfree aspects of the pseudo-contract mean that many may not comply. They then will have only the family to rely upon – if they have one. I do indeed believe that the metaphor of the state as the ultimate safety net or as 'the last resort' has become false. When the state starts to withdraw from its responsibilities, the net is safe no more. The family is becoming the last resort that picks up the pieces of a fragmented welfare system. It will obviously become seriously overburdened financially, physically and emotionally, but this seldom becomes a public concern. The last step on this road is total disaffiliation.

Those abandoned by all the public institutions and who have no family are left out in the cold. This may happen everywhere albeit it occurs more often in poorer countries or countries less attentive to the norms or recommendations of 'European' bodies.

An uncertain conclusion

Human relations are complex. One of the manifestations of this complexity is that there have always been many – historically changing – ways of getting access to resources. A precise accounting of giving and getting may be instrumental in modern business. Human relationships, however, cannot be reduced to book-keeping even if many of them contain an economic kernel. Moreover, as a rule they cannot be governed by the high risk activities of the stock exchange or the casino.

Conceptual clarity, the separation of relatively clear principles, is a legitimate exercise. Reality is different, though. Bread and dignity, freedom and security are shared needs. When bread is available under humiliating conditions and dignity is guaranteed by law on an empty stomach, the need for a dignified meal cannot be satisfied.

I have argued that modern social contracts, the labour contract and social insurance, offer socially relatively fair and legitimate instruments to societal policy: they represent successful attempts to assure dignified meals for many. These messy contracts can incorporate opposed interests and to some extent reconcile indi-vidualism with collective structures. This has been the basis of their strong civil support and relative stability: the 'apparent inconsistencies' have indeed become a 'source of stability' (Marshall 1965: 164). This stability is being now questioned and shaken.

The criticism has to be accepted that the socially advantageous features of messy contracts have been limited to those covered by them. This limitation may become increasingly unjust as their coverage is shrinking following the restructuring of the labour market. Many propose giving up messy contracts – besides the other reasons already discussed – because of this failure.

Yet, so far globalization has carried with it increasing inequalities, increasing insecurities and anxieties, and increasing poverty. The old systems of social protection may not be adaptable to a new social landscape built on quicksand. The current functional alternatives – the insurance market with its inevitable failures, charity with all its non-democratic potentials, and the escalating criminalization of poverty – do not augur well. Protective functions will not be realized without 'messy' constructs accepting, among others, the principles of social solidarity and social rights. Whether national and global civil society will re-discover and re-endorse these values, and whether global capital will allow their rediscovery and re-endorsement is uncertain. Without them, however, there is little hope for the creation of defences against insecurities, and ultimately against the erosion of freedoms.

Notes

1 The chapter is a reworked version of a conference paper given first in 1997. I gratefully acknowledge the encouragement of S.M. (Mike) Miller, and the helpful comments of Michael Adler, Paddy Baron, Balazs Krémer, Dorothy and Adrian Sinfield and Guy Standing. A previous version of the paper was published as Ferge 2000.
2 The classical representatives of the social contract tradition are Hobbes, Locke, Rousseau and Kant (Gough 1957). The contract view lives on in modern philosophy, the work of John Rawls being the best known example (Rawls 1971). The concept of the social contract has acquired pragmatic albeit symbolic connotations in the second half of the twentieth century, particularly in continental Europe. The need for a new or renewed social contract usually occurs during or after turbulent times.
3 Bolderson and Mabbett (1995) argue in a similar vein about the advantages of social security 'mongrels' that incorporate different 'allocative principles'. Unfortunately I came across their paper too late to make full use of it. I borrow their expression, however. My own concept, the 'legitimate and legitimating principle of access to resources' may be closer to my meaning, but it is clumsy.
4 Lawrence Mead (1985) argued that even rights-based benefits left poor people 'in the position of petitioners, dependent on society's goodwill, as anyone who possesses only rights' (quoted in Walter 1989: 74).
5 The revocation of so-called 'positive' rights would become more difficult if they were also enshrined in constitutions, similar to negative rights. This, however, is a highly contested issue (Sunstein 1994). The European Charter of Fundamental Human Rights now under debate in the EU aims at making the rights already incorporated in the various charters broader and more legally enforceable.
6 For a more detailed discussion of 'black and white lies' see Ferge (2000).
7 The now widely accepted refundable income tax credit has good points, but it weakens the claim for a living wage.
8 Even if the framework continues to exist, the eligibility rules are tightened, the periods covered are shortened, the rates of the benefit are reduced, and the work-tests are made harsher in many countries.

References

Atkinson, A.B. (1998) 'Social exclusion, poverty and unemployment', in A.B. Atkinson and J. Hills (eds), *Exclusion, Employment and Opportunity*, STICERD CASE Paper 4, London: Centre for Analysis of Social Exclusion, London School of Economics, pp.1–20.

Baldwin, P. (1990) *The Politics of Social Solidarity: Class Bases of the European Welfare State 1875–1975*, Cambridge, New York: Cambridge University Press.

Bolderson, H. and Mabbett, D. (1995) 'Mongrels and thoroughbreds: A cross-national look at social security systems', *European Journal of Policy Research* 28: 119–139.

Boyer, R. and Drache, D. (1996) *States Against Markets. The Limits of Globalization*, London and New York: Routledge.

Castel, R. (1995) *Les métamorphoses de la question sociale. Une chronique du salariat*, Paris: Fayard.

Dollard, D. and Kraay, A. (2000) *Growth is Good for the Poor*, Development Research Group, The World Bank, March 2000.

Emanuel, H. (1998) 'Controlling admissions and stays in social security programs', in P.R. de Jong and T.R. Marmor (eds) *Social Policy and the Labour Market*, International Studies on Social Security, FISS. vol. 2, Aldershot, Brookfield, Singapore, Sidney: Ashgate, pp. 161–72.

Eriksen, T. and Palmer, E. (1997) 'The concept of work capacity', in P.R. de Jong and T.R. Marmor (eds) *Social Policy and the Labour Market*, International Studies on Social Security, FISS. vol. 2, Aldershot, Brookfield, Singapore, Sidney: Ashgate, pp. 149–60.

Ferge, Zsuzsa (2000) 'In Defence of Messy or Multi-Principle Contracts', *European Journal of Social Security*, vol. 2, no. 1, pp. 7–33.

Fried, C. (1981) *Contract as Promise: A Theory of Contractual Obligation*, Cambridge: Harvard University Press.

Gerth, H.H. and Mills, C.W. (eds) (1946) *From Max Weber: Essays in Sociology*, New York: Oxford University Press.

Goodin, R.E. (1998) 'More than anyone bargained for: Beyond the welfare contract', *Ethics and International Affairs*, vol. 12, pp. 141–58.

Gough, J.W. (1957) *The Social Contract*, Oxford: The Clarendon Press.

Holzmann, R. and Jorgensen, S. (2000) *Social Risk Management: A New Conceptual Framework for Social Protection and Beyond*, SP Discussion Paper No.0006, The World Bank.

Issing, O. (1998) 'Der Sozialstaat auf der Prüfstand', in K. Morath (ed.) *Verlässliche soziale Sicherung*, Bad-Homburg: Frankfurter Institut – Stiftung Marktwirtschaft und Politik, pp. 13–19.

Lockwood, D. (1964) 'Social integration and system integration', in G.K. Zollschan and W. Hirsch (eds), *Explorations in Social Change*, Boston: Houghton Mifflin Company.

Marshall, T.H. (1965) *Class, Citizenship, and Social Development*, New York: Anchor Books Edition.

Mead, L. (1985) *Beyond Entitlement: The Social Obligations of Citizenship*, New York: Free Press.

Polanyi, K. (1944) *The Great Transformation*, Boston: Beacon Press.

Rawls, J. (1971) *A Theory of Justice*, Cambridge, Mass: The Belknap Press of Harvard University Press.

Rhys-Williams, J. (1942) *Something to Look Forward To*, London: Macdonald.

Sen, A. (2000) *Social Exclusion: Concept, Application and Scrutiny*, Manila: Office of Environment and Development, Asian Development Bank.

Standing, G. (1999) *Global Labour Flexibility: Seeking Distributive Justice*, London: Macmillan Press Ltd.

Sunstein, C. (1994) Against Positive Rights. Paper presented at the Conference on The Meaning of Rights in Post-Communism, Central European University, Budapest, June.

Supiot, A. (1995) 'L'avenir d'un vieux couple: travail et sécurité sociale', *Droit Social*, no. 9–10, Septembre–Octobre.

Swaan, A. de (1988) *In Care of the State: Health Care, Education and Welfare in Europe and the USA in the Modern Era*, Oxford/New York: Oxford University Press/Polity Press.

van Parijs, P. (1995) *Real Freedom for All: What (If Anything) Can Justify Capitalism?*, Oxford: Clarendon Press.

Veit-Wilson, J. (1998). *Setting Adequacy Standards: How Governments Define Minimum Incomes*, Bristol: The Policy Press.

Walter, T. (1989) *Basic Income: Freedom From Poverty, Freedom to Work*, London, New York: Marion Boyars.

World Bank Policy Research Report (1994) *Averting the Old Age Crisis: Policies to Protect the Old and Promote Growth*, New York: Oxford University Press.

World Bank (1995) *Hungary: Structural Reforms for Sustainable Growth*, A World Bank Country Study, Washington D.C.: The World Bank.

Chapter 4

Live and let love?

Reflections on the unfinished sexual revolution of our times

Jeffrey Weeks

Sexual insecurity and social policy

At the centre of contemporary insecurities is an uncertainty over the representation and meaning of sexuality. Despite the celebration of choice and diversity supposedly intrinsic to the late modern world, gender and sexuality remain battlegrounds of contested meanings. We may acknowledge the fact of sexual diversity, but we find it difficult to value it. Boundaries of taste and tolerance may crumble, but are then drawn and redrawn as we try to demarcate the lines between appropriate and inappropriate, 'right' and 'wrong' behaviour. Sexual imagery may play throughout our culture in books, the media, advertising. Religion, medicine, psychology, sociology, history and biology may discourse endlessly about the implications of sexual change. There may be an unprecedented volubility about the erotic in everyday life. Yet it is not too extreme to say that we continue to dwell in a state of sexual insecurity, despite, or because of, the 'sexual revolution' of our time. This poses immense challenges, not least for those foolhardy enough to attempt to regulate, or shape policies towards, sexual change.

The 'sexual revolution' has been widely discussed, applauded and execrated since the 1960s. It has been hailed as setting the agenda for what Roy Jenkins called a 'civilised society' (see Weeks 1981/1989: 243), and as the harbinger of the 'great disruption' which has undermined Western values of trust (Fukuyama 1999). Yet apparently simple moves towards formalizing the legal equality of, for example, non-heterosexual people, become symbolic testing grounds that can humble even the strongest of governments. The mighty 1997 Labour Government in Britain, the first ever to commit itself (in however qualified a form) to equality of treatment of homosexuals, finds its modest moves to equalize the age of consent, and to remove discriminatory legislation (such as 'Clause 28', which prevents the 'promotion by local government of homosexuality') legislatively blocked as the 'forces of conservatism' mobilize their formidable remaining energies (see Epstein *et al.* 2000). Some revolution, many might think. The revolution is clearly unfinished.

But that seems to be the fate of attempts to change beliefs, behaviours and attitudes towards sexuality, whether by ostentatiously attempting to go backwards, to 'restore traditional values', or by seeking a new sexual order. There is no simple linear history of progress towards greater toleration and individual freedom; nor, of course, of collapse into 'moral decline', that much spoken of but little defined concept. Instead there are local battles, symbolic moments, moral panics, infinitesimal shifts, moves forward and back. Sometimes great crusades push in one direction. Public apathy may push in another. Governments might will an end; but the unexpected, unanticipated consequences are just as likely to shift the reality on the ground or in the bedroom. Sexuality may be peculiarly susceptible to socio-cultural moulding, as Gagnon and Simon (1974) suggested. But it rarely changes to plan, will or statutory instruction.

That makes the formulation of policy towards the sexual sphere fraught, hazardous and usually unrewarding. Since the churches largely ceded the lead to states in shaping the regulation of sexual behaviour (a long drawn out, and still not fully completed process, gathering pace in the nineteenth century, galloping up the hill in the later part of the twentieth), governments, especially in Britain, have often shuffled away from direct responsibility. Governmental bodies, national and local, have happily intervened to control the prostitute, but have fought shy of banning prostitution. Single parents have been the focus of many panics and much moralizing, but promiscuity, adultery and pre-marital sex have not been banned. The ideal of heterosexual marriage might be lauded, and its decline richly lamented, but social engineering to entrench 'the traditional family' has rarely been attempted. The 1960s may have given birth to a notable series of progressive reforms – on censorship, divorce, abortion, homosexuality – but these were the products of 'private conscience' initiatives (and discreet government support) rather than public beneficence. The 'dangerous sexualities', which Mort (1987) acutely analysed, have often tested the moral enthusiasms of even the most evangelical of politicians, alert to the dangers to their own standing and ambitions – not to mention their own private lives.

Yet sexuality, implicitly or explicitly, has been at the heart of social policy for a very long time, because it raises profound questions about the social order. If we look at the key moments in British history since at least the beginning of the nineteenth century we see that in one way or another a preoccupation with sexual behaviour has been central to them (see Weeks 1981/1989, on which the following discussion is based). In the crisis of the French revolutionary wars in the early century we see a concern with moral decline which, it was believed, was integral to the collapse of the ancient regime. Middle class ideologues sought a new bourgeois morality to challenge the immorality of the aristocracy and the amorality of the labouring masses. In the 1830s and 1840s, with the first crisis of the new industrial order, there was a near obsessive interest in the sexuality of working women, and of children working in the mines and factories. The great series of Royal Commissions of the period reported in detail on the sexual licence of the new manufacturing centres. By the mid nineteenth century, fuelled by the spread of epidemics such as cholera and typhoid in the overcrowded towns and cities, attempts to reform society concentrated on questions of health and personal morality. From the 1860s to the 1890s, prostitution, venereal disease, public immorality and private vice were at the heart of debate, many choosing to see in moral decay a symbol of imperial decay.

Such preoccupations were not unique to the nineteenth century. If anything, sexuality became more and more a public obsession, in the twentieth, particularly in relation to the integrity of the British population, which in turn fed into the origins of the welfare state. In the years before the First World War, there was a vogue for eugenics amongst social reformers, the planned breeding of the best. Though never dominant, it had a significant influence in shaping welfare policies and the attempt to reorder national priorities in the face of international competition. It also fed into a burgeoning racism in the inter-war years as politicians feared a declining population which would give dominance to 'inferior races'. Into the 1940s, the key moment in the establishment of the Welfare State, there was an urgent concern with the merits of birth control ('family planning') in ensuring that the right sort of people built families, and of the appropriate roles of men and women (especially women) in the family in the brave new world of social democracy. We should not forget that the great social policy theorist, Richard Titmuss, was using eugenic language as late as the 1940s (Weeks 1981/1989: 234); and it has recently come to light that the very model of social democracy, Sweden, continued covertly to pursue eugenic policies to sterilize the mentally unfit into the 1970s (Boyes 2000: 19). Linked with this, in the depth of the Cold War, there was a new searching out of sexual degenerates, especially homosexuals, who not only lived outside families but were also, apparently, peculiarly susceptible to treason.

The climate may change, but the questions of social order remain to the fore. By the 1960s, a new liberalism ('permissiveness') seemed torn between relaxing the old authoritarian social codes and finding new modes of social regulation, based on the latest in social psychology and a redefinition of the public/private divide (Weeks 1981/1989). During the 1970s and 1980s there was in effect the beginnings of a backlash against what were seen as the excesses of the earlier decade, and perhaps for the first time sexuality became an explicit front-line political issue as the emergence of the New Right targeted the 'decline of the family', feminism and the new homosexual militancy as potent symbols of national decline (Durham 1997). These dramatically unsuccessful policies – by the 1990s there were more divorces, more unmarried mothers, fewer marriages, a higher incidence of co-habitation, more open homosexuality than ever before – set the scene for the more explicit sexual policies of the present, with the idea of 'sexual citizenship' for the first time an explicit, if still contested, item on the policy agenda (Weeks 1998; 2000, chapter 12). What was covert has left its closet; what was latent has become blatant. But the anxieties about the relation of sexuality to wider social concerns remain high. The dramatic escalation of fear and loathing concerning child sex abuse in the summer of 2000, fuelled by a particularly horrific murder of a young girl, illustrates the ways in which the figure of the 'pervert' in the form of 'the paedophile' can become the focus of a complex set of social fears – from abuse of authority to widespread anxiety about crime and the condition of poor and neglected housing estates (see the British press, *passim*, throughout July and August 2000).

Clearly a number of different but related concerns are present in these recurrent debates about morality and sexual behaviour: the relations between men and women, the problem of sexual deviance, the question of family and other relationships, the relations between adults and children, and the issue of difference, whether of class, gender or race. Each of these has a long history, but in the past couple of hundred years they have become increasingly central concerns, with their sexual implications well to the fore. They illustrate the power of the belief that debates about sexuality are debates about the nature of society: as sex goes, so goes society; but similarly, as society goes, so goes sexuality.

Remaking sexuality

What we term 'sexuality', a 'historic construct' in Foucault's (1979) famous, if mistranslated phrase, is shaped in and through such debates, social interventions – and the complex resistances they engender. Sexuality is a product of both structure and agency. We make sexual history, as much as sexuality makes us (Weeks 2000).

What is remarkable about the past generation, I want to suggest, is the extent to which sexuality has been remade: not for everyone at the same pace, or to the same effect, but no-one has escaped this long revolution. We can note the necessary reservations. National surveys still tell us that on the whole the British population is more conservative than many think (Wellings *et al.* 1994). Most people still marry, and re-marry, even if divorce is high. The average number of partners is still decently low. Serial monogamy is the norm. Cohabitation before marriage may now be routine, but most offspring of such unions are still registered by both parents. Homosexuality may be more tolerated, but most lesbians or gays still feel constrained in coming out, and the legal situation remains, despite the best efforts of many committed campaigners, inequitable. I could go on. It is an unfinished revolution, working its way through the interstices of everyday life in an uneven way. Nevertheless, it would be foolhardy not to recognize what has changed, at a remarkable pace in historic terms.

I shall not argue that the results of all the changes that have taken place are an unalloyed success. There are victims as well as gainers from the changes. Sexuality in itself is neither good nor bad, but a potentiality for pain as much as pleasure, risk as well as satisfaction. But anyone who has lived through the period since 1945, the period of the triumph of welfarism, can be in no doubt of the significance of the changes that have taken place. One of the reasons why assorted campaigns to 'turn back the clock', go 'back to basics' and restore 'traditional values' rarely find much of a toe-hold on general public consciousness is that no-one, not even the most ardent advocates of a sexual counter-revolution, is immune from the effects of change. Which family does not have an unmarried mother, an out-of-the-closet homosexual, a divorced relative, within its bosom? Things have gone too far for a simple return to a traditional past (a past which in any case is pretty mythical). We are in the midst of a long, unfinished, but a permanent revolution, and on a global scale – which makes for a profound sense of uncertainty, but also for unheard of opportunities.

It is in this context that new claims to citizenship – 'sexual' or 'intimate' citizenship (Plummer 1995) – have arisen. Plummer has discussed new claims for citizenship in relation to what he describes as new 'sexual stories'. Human beings, he argues, are inveterate storytellers, and societies may be seen as webs of stories and narratives which through their interaction bind us together. New stories emerge when there are people ready to listen to and understand them through interpretive communities. The new stories about gender, sexuality and the body which have been told since the 1960s have been possible because of the emergence of new movements and communities that both give rise to and circulate and rewrite these stories. The most common narratives are stories which tell of discrimination, prejudice and empowerment, stories which tell of coming out as lesbian and gay or as a strong, independent woman, stories of victimization and of survival, stories of difference and of similarity, stories of identity and stories of relationships. These new stories about the self, about sexuality and gender, are the context for the emergence of the would be sexual citizen because these stories telling of exclusion, through gender, sexuality, race, bodily appearance or function, have as their corollary the demand for inclusion: for equal rights under the law, in politics, in economics, in social matters and in sexual matters. They pose questions about who should control our bodies, the limits of the body, the burden of custom and of the state. They are stories which spring up from everyday life, but in turn place new demands on the wider community for the development of more responsive policies, in economics, welfare, the law, culture.

In the case of AIDS, people living with devastating illness have taken the lead in defining both medical practice and caring relationships (Epstein 1996). Non-heterosexuals have challenged the hegemony of patterns of marriage by demanding partnership rights or same sex marriages (Sullivan 1997). Counter-discourses, oppositional knowledges, grassroots politics and self-activity have undermined traditional political forms, and begun to define new agendas. There has been an accumulation of new social and cultural capital, where new voices, new collective subjectivities have put forward their claims through a variety of social and political practices (Blasius 1994; Weeks and Holland 1996).

New forms, new values, new forms of recognition have to be struggled for, often against fierce opposition representing traditional (or more likely, neo-traditional) values. In recent years we have seen the rise of new fundamentalisms, whether embodied in the Christian right in the United States (see, for example, Herman 1997), or in various transnational political religious identities – Islamic fundamentalism, Hindu revivalism and so on (Bhatt 1997). Concerns with the body, differentiation between men and women, and sexual identity are central to these movements. Nor is fundamentalism, which Giddens (1994) has described as a refusal of dialogue, a refusal to recognise diversity and difference, confined to religion. Various forms of fundamentalism have been manifest in the new social movements as much as in the old social forms, as the 'sex wars' over differing interpretations of feminism in the United States dismally confirm (see Duggan and Hunter 1995). The new pluralism can itself become a new form of fundamentalism if we believe that every distinct identity and community must be marked off by wars and barbed wire from another. The challenge of the late modern world is not to find a new unitary system of values, or to retreat into a hard won new identity, but rather to balance diversity with common values. This is what the argument for sexual or intimate citizenship is ultimately about. New forms of citizenship must accommodate the real changes which are undermining traditional patterns of being, and of legitimacy: transformations of intimate life; the rise of new forms of individualism; and the pluralization of life forms. The remainder of my discussion will focus on these themes.

Transformations

We have, of course, in some ways been here before. As Durkheim noted at the beginning of the twentieth century, in terms which many could have echoed a century later:

> Today traditional morality is shaken and no other has been brought forward to replace it. The older duties have lost their power without our being able to see clearly and with assurance where our new duties lie. Different minds hold opposed ideas and we are passing through a period of crisis. It is not then surprising that we do not feel the pressure of moral rules as they were felt in the past. They cannot appear to us in their old majesty, since they are practically non-existent.
>
> (Durkheim 1974: 68–9)

Just as changes in the late nineteenth and early twentieth centuries were responses to the unsettling of all relationships in the wake of unprecedented changes posed by the impact of industrialization, urbanization, and the uneven process of democratization, so today we can observe features which are products of a distinctive conjuncture as the juggernaut of modernity (Giddens 1990) grinds on. We are witnessing the effects of the two closely interrelated tendencies which, I suggest, are crucial: 'detraditionalization' and 'the transformation of intimacy' (compare Giddens 1992, 1994; Weeks 1998), both of which can be linked to the contested, but undeniable, process of globalization.

Throughout the western world we are witnessing a breakdown of traditional forms and values, as rapid economic, social and cultural changes on a global scale undermine many of the traditional bastions of legitimate authority (for a summary argument see Giddens 1994; Beck and Beck-Gernsheim 1995). If we look at the role of the churches, customary patterns of life, state forms, and the family, we can see profound shifts of belief and attitudes (for a more detailed discussion see Weeks 2000, chapter 12). The traditional ordered distinctions and balances between men and women have been radically challenged by both material and cultural changes, not least the impact of feminism, and the changing role of women in the workforce. The binary divide between homosexuality and heterosexuality, which was codified in the nineteenth century and has come to be regarded as the very definition of natural in the twentieth century, has been significantly challenged by the public emergence of vocal lesbian and gay movements and collective identities. In the wake of these movements a more radical sexual fringe has emerged, 'queering' sexuality in new ways (Weeks 1985; Evans 1993; Plummer 1995). The relationship between adults and children has become particularly fraught, the subject of constant negotiation and renegotiation, as a succession of moral panics and public controversies, latterly represented by the epidemic of sexual abuse accounts, and the endemic threat of paedophilia, dramatize our fears and inconsistencies.

In this context it is easy to note many of the symptoms of breakdown in the traditional patterns of domestic life. The divorce figures, the incidence of single parenting, the delay of marriage, the rise of cohabitation, a rapid rise of single households, the emergence of new patterns of intimacy, such as lesbian and gay 'families of choice', all these are indices of profound change. At the same time the balance between private life and public life is being constantly renegotiated. What was hitherto regarded as the most intimate sphere has now become a major topic of public concern. Contrariwise, what we had always regarded as the legitimate sphere of public concern – the quality of life, the nature of public services, safety on the streets – has in many Western countries as a result of radical right policies increasingly been subject to privatization (Weeks 1995).

The pessimists, such as Fukuyama (1999) regard these changes with the deepest gloom. Communitarians such as Etzioni (1995) look forward to the bolstering of family life, even if in new forms. The optimists detect new opportunities for 'life experiments' (see Giddens 1992; Beck and Beck-Gernsheim 1995; Weeks, Donovan and Heaphy 1999). But whatever the ethical stance we take, and whatever the necessary qualifications we make, such as those cited above, there can be little doubt of massive, irreversible, shifts in the inherited patterns of intimate life. And whatever the difficulties, and continuing patterns of inequality, violence and struggle, it has often been women who have been in the vanguard of these changes. In Britain, for example, most divorces are initiated by women (though whether this is a flight to freedom, or an enforced escape from oppression is contested: see Jamieson 1998).

These changes are related in turn to what Anthony Giddens (1992) has called 'the transformation of intimacy', a long-term shift towards the ideal of the democratic egalitarian relationship between men and women, men and men, women and women. We need not argue that the ideal is a reality in all or perhaps even a majority of relationships. The empirical evidence underlines the persistence of inherited inequalities between men and women, as young people reproduce the sexual brutalities and struggles that optimists hoped had long disappeared, and older ones slip complacently into conventional patterns (Jamieson 1998; Holland *et al.* 1998). Yet the same evidence suggests a widespread acceptance of the merits of companionate and more equal relationships, even as we fail to achieve them. The egalitarian relationship has become a measure by which increasing numbers of people feel they must judge their own individual lives. At the centre of this ideal is the fundamental belief that love relationships and partnerships should be a matter not of arrangement or tradition, but of personal choice, based on a balance of attraction, desire, mutual trust and compatibility. This inevitably introduces a new element of contingency into intimate life. Although the ideal may still be lifelong commitments, many people stay together only so long as the relationship fulfills the needs of the partners.

But there is compelling evidence that this is being balanced by a changing, but not necessarily weaker, ideal of commitment based on negotiation. Ties of obligation, based on blood relationship, or formal ties, are increasingly being displaced by ideas of commitments that have to be worked out day by day, week by week. As Finch and Mason (1993) have argued in relationship to kinship relationships in contemporary Britain, people still feel bound by ties of commitment to blood relatives, but these are subject all the time to negotiation. In research on non-heterosexual families of choice in Britain (see Weeks, Donovan and Heaphy, 1998, 1999), it has become clear, amongst self-defined non-heterosexual people at least, that the language of obligation and duty is being displaced by a language of negotiated commitment and mutual responsibility.

This need not, should not, mean a minimization of commitment. On the contrary, because relationships are developed on the basis of choice rather than ascription, they are potentially stronger because they are freely chosen. Our research (Weeks, Donovan and Heaphy, 1998, 1999) suggests that new patterns of relationships are no less strong in caring for children or the vulnerable whether young or old. Commitments to mutual care, responsibility and respect are at the heart of these elective relationships. My point is, however, that these represent a significant shift away from the sorts of duties and obligations that tied people together in the past.

These patterns are not, of course, universal. There is strong evidence that the achievement of egalitarian relationships is in fact more likely outside heterosexual relationships (Giddens 1992; Dunne 1997; Jamieson 1998). The inherited inequalities between the genders are constantly reproduced in the intimate as well as other spheres, as much research as well as our day-to-day experience underlines. But the urge to equality is now, I suggest, at the centre of increasing numbers of relationships, however inadequately it may be realized.

Autonomy

These new patterns may be seen as examples of a new, or accentuated, individualism in Western cultures. There can be no doubt that the economic and cultural changes of the past twenty or thirty years have tended to exalt the individual over the collective. The sweep of economic liberalism throughout most Western countries since the 1970s has elevated individual self-expression and material well-being and undermined many of the traditional sources of solidarity such as the trade unions and other collective forms. The paradox of the 1980s in countries like Britain and the United States was that an extreme economic individualism coincided with attempts at social authoritarianism: at restoring traditional values, the traditional family, tightening the barriers against radical change (Weeks 1995). The 1990s demonstrated, however, that the triumph of economic individualism has tended to undermine the social authoritarianism, and given rise to a new libertarianism where anything potentially goes. It is one of the more interesting sights of the recent turbulence of conservatism in Britain that some right-wing thinkers who ten years ago would have been in the vanguard of social authoritarianism are now justifying the decriminalization of drugs, lesbian and gay marriages, and forms of sexual hedonism. The idea of individual freedom cannot be confined to one sphere; it interpenetrates all, dissolving traditional bonds and producing a new 'moral fluency' with incalculable consequences (see Mulgan 1997).

But anything goes libertarianism is not the only possibility. I suggest that equally likely are the emergence of new forms of what I would describe as 'democratic autonomy' (Weeks 1995). The principles of democratic autonomy suggest the need both for individual fulfilment and for mutual involvement, and there are many examples one could cite of this being worked through in practice. I will give one example, but an example which I think throws light on the whole transformation of relationships that is taking place: the HIV/AIDS crisis. As we know, the first manifestations of the crisis were in the gay communities of North America and later of Europe, which have been characterized as the very exemplars of sexual hedonism. And there can be no doubt that the easy sexual interactions of the gay culture of the west coast or New York did help the rapid spread of the HIV virus within the gay community. But the most striking feature of the response to the epidemic from the gay community was the way in which it brought out a new culture of responsibility, for the self and for others (Weeks 1995). The discourse of safer sex is precisely about balancing individual needs and responsibility to others in a community of identity whose organizing principle is the avoidance of infection and the provision of mutual support. The sexual ties of the new gay cultures of Western society proved to be strongly imagined community ties which produced a massive effort of collective self-activity in developing community based responses to HIV and AIDS, which showed the way forward for publicly funded services in Britain and elsewhere (Adam 1992; Weeks 1995). But in turn AIDS has raised complex issues about citizenship, and especially about the degree to which the execrated person with a life threatening syndrome who nevertheless fails to engage in 'safer sex' can be fully included in the social (see for example Watney 1994; Woodhead 1998).

New forms of mutual responsibility and autonomy are also manifest in what I have described as families of choice, the varied patterns of domestic involvement, sexual intimacy and mutual responsibilities that are increasingly displacing traditional patterns of marriage and the family (Weston 1991; Blasius 1994; Weeks, Donovan and Heaphy 1999). All these, I would suggest, are examples of what Giddens (1992) calls 'experiments in living' which many of us in late modern societies are forced to engage in. There are, of course, constraints – economic, social cultural, personal – which severely limit free choice. It is easier for some people to adopt different lifestyles than others. Many are still trapped in patterns of exclusion and poverty. Yet traditional ways of life are no longer viable or meaningful for very many people, who have no choice but to choose. They have to find ways of living together which are meaningful for them. For many that is a profoundly fear-making threat; for others it is an opportunity for inventing themselves afresh.

Diversity

Greater individualization has to be associated with a wider acceptance of diversity, in life choices and in identity. Just as detraditionalization destabilizes traditional patterns of relationships, so traditional concepts of the self and individual and collective identities are fundamentally undermined. Increasingly today, identity is not something you assume or are born into or have to remain fixed with all your life. It is something that you make for yourself, as part of what has been called the 'reflexive project of the self' (Giddens 1991). We can no longer assume, either, a single identity from which all social action proceeds. We have multiple possible identities – as men or women, black or white, straight or gay, Welsh, British, European, or whatever – each of which carries different, and often contradictory, loyalties, claims and commitments. Identities are varied and changing. We can no longer regard ourselves as one thing throughout all our lives. Identities are 'projects', 'narrative quests', 'performances' (Giddens 1991; Butler 1990; Garber 1992). We are hybrids (Bhabha 1990; Sinfield 1997). This does not mean a dissolution of the self, but a recognition that the task of finding an anchor for the self, a narrative which gives meaning to all our disparate potential belongings, is a task of invention and of self-invention (Plummer 1995).

Post-structuralist and post-modernist questionings of the enlightenment myth of the unitary self have opened up a whole series of questions. What is it, for instance, that gives unity to the self? For Michel Foucault it is in an important sense about being an artist of the self, creating an aesthetics of your own life (Foucault 1988). Others, like Agnes Heller (1984), have raised critical questions about what constitutes a meaningful life, how we balance a strong sense of ourselves with the involvement with significant others which alone makes our lives have meaning. These are profoundly important issues concerning ethics and values, and in a very real sense the post-modernist challenge has led not to an abandonment of a quest for meaning, but on the contrary a search for meaning, a meaning, however, that is constructed by us and not for us in some hidden heaven (Weeks 1995).

The question of the nature of the self is not simply a product of wild surmise and theoretical speculation (Melucci 1996). Globalization has dissolved many of the differences between cultures at the same time as it has reinforced new particularisms. New technologies have fundamentally questioned the fixity of our sense of self and of body. Reproductive technologies have made it possible to bypass the traditional human processes in the creation of new individuals. A new obsession with health and fitness has led to a refashioning of the body along new lines. Cosmetic surgery can remake the body from the size of one's breasts to the shape of one's nose, from the colour of one's hair to the pigmentation of one's skin. Genetic engineering opens possibilities for choosing the sex of one's offspring, eliminating those with inherited diseases, eliminating the unfit, even, if we accept the wilder eyed enthusiasts, eventually choosing our sexual orientation. The revolution in information technology represented by the Internet opens new opportunities for communication of desire, for representation of the body, and for sexual interaction (Wolmark 1999). The body itself has become a reflexive project, no longer the fixed point on which identity is built, but something to be made and remade through the maze of shifting potential identities. The women's movement and the lesbian and gay movements of the past thirty years have done more than simply reflect pre-existing identities. They have helped to make new identities possible through their collective experiences. They have provided a focus of meaning. In turn, of course, they pose fundamental questions about politics, cultural belonging and personal needs (see, for example, Cooper 1995).

These new subjectivities and identities are cultural creations. They provide individual and collective narratives through which we make sense of new circum-stances and new possibilities. They are the 'necessary fictions' through which we negotiate the hazards of everyday life in a world in a process of constant change (Weeks 1995). And in turn they give sustenance to the new claims to citizenship.

Citizenship

Most discussion on citizenship has followed Marshall (1950) in concentrating on three particular phases: the civil or legal, the political and the social. Contemporary critiques and developments of the idea of citizenship have demonstrated the lacunae in Marshall's teleology: by broadening the scope (Andrews 1991; Turner 1993); uncovering the gendered nature of the concept (Walby 1994; Lister 1996, 1997; *Feminist Review* 1997); and laying bare its national and racialized dimensions (Anthias and Yuval-Davis 1992). It is now apparent that the citizenship discourse embraces a multiplicity of interlocked strands which reveal the dense inter-connections of class, gender – and sexuality.

Assumptions about sexuality have always been implicit in the discourse of citizenship, but those assumptions have traditionally been narrowly familial, heterosexual and normative. The claim to sexual citizenship is a claim for the incorporation of issues which have hitherto been occluded or excluded. Sexual, or intimate, citizenship is about the *control (or not) over* one's body, feelings, relationships: *access (or not) to* representations, relationships, public spaces, etc.; and *socially grounded choices (or not) about* identities, gender experiences.

(Plummer 1995: 151; his emphasis)

It is a sensitizing concept, which alerts us to new concerns, hitherto marginalized in public discourse: with the body, its possibilities, needs and pleasures; with new sexualized identities; and with the forces that inhibit their free, consensual development in a democratic polity committed to full and equal citizenship (for overviews of the debates see Evans 1993, 1995; Richardson 1998; Bell and Binnie 2000). It has a positive content, in the articulation of new claims to rights and 'sexual justice' (Kaplan 1997). But it also offers a sharp critique of traditional discourses on citizenship, and on the limitations of contemporary debates.

The would-be sexual citizen exists because of the new primacy given to sexual subjectivity in the contemporary world. The claim to a new form of belonging, which is what citizenship is ultimately about, arises from and reflects the remaking of the self and the multiplicity and diversity of possible identities that characterize the late, or post, modern world. The would-be sexual citizen, despite obvious traceable precursors in a complex past, is a new presence because of ever accelerating transformations of everyday life, and the social and political implications that flow from this. Which is why the sexual citizen deserves more serious attention than s/he has previously received: this new personage is a harbinger of a new politics of intimacy and everyday life.

Even thirty years or so ago, no one would have said, for example, 'I am gay/ lesbian', or 'sadomasochist', or 'transgendered', or 'queer', or anything like that as a defining characteristic of personhood and of social involvement and presence. Today, at least in the metropolitan heartlands of Western societies, it is commonplace for many previously marginalized people – those belonging to sexual minorities – to define themselves both in terms of personal and collective identities by their sexual attributes, and to claim recognition, rights and respect as a consequence.

I have argued elsewhere (Weeks 1995) that the new sexual movements of the past generation, particularly feminism and the lesbian and gay movement, have had two characteristic elements: a moment of transgression, and a moment of citizenship. The moment of transgression is characterized by the constant invention and re-invention of new senses of the self, and new challenges to the inherited institutions and traditions that hitherto had excluded these new subjects: the moment when the non-heterosexual comes out as lesbian or gay, rejecting the negative stereotypes; when the housewife joins a consciousness raising group and redefines herself as a feminist, when the cross dresser proclaims him or herself as transgendered, when the marginally different or the apparently normatively ordinary becomes 'queer'. The characteristic form of expression is subversive of traditional ways of being: the public demonstrations, the camaraderie of collective political action, the new forms of self expression – the men dressed as nuns, the mythologized bra-burning of feminists, the women in leather on motorbikes in the vanguard of lesbian and gay pride marches, the kiss-ins in public spaces in capital cities. The aim of such carnivalesque displays, whether conscious or not, is to challenge the status quo and various forms of social exclusion by exotic manifestations of difference.

Yet contained within these movements is also a claim to inclusion, to the acceptance of diversity, and a recognition of and respect for alternative ways of being, to a broadening of the definition of belonging. This is the moment of citizenship: the claim to equal protection of the law, to equal rights in employment, parenting, social status, access to welfare provision, and partnerships rights, or even marriage, for same sex couples (Donovan, Heaphy and Weeks 2000).

Although these tend to be different moments in the discourse of sexual politics, they are, I would suggest, both necessary to each other. Without the transgressive moment, the claims of the hitherto excluded would barely be noticed in the apparently rigid and complacent structures of old and well entrenched societies. Transgression appears necessary to face the status quo with its inadequacies, to hold a mirror up to its prejudices and fears. But without the claim to full citizenship, difference can never find a recognized place. The sexual citizen then makes a claim to transcend the limits of the personal sphere by going public, but the going public is, in a necessary but nevertheless paradoxical move, about protecting the possibilities of private life and private choice in a more inclusive society.

The notion of sexual or intimate citizenship, then, is an attempt to remedy the limitations of earlier notions of citizenship, to make the concept more comprehensive. But it simultaneously requires us to accommodate different analytical categories: not only class, not even just gender and race, but also the impact of the heterosexual/ homosexual binarism, the institutionalization of heterosexuality, and the question of equity and justice for emergent 'sexual minorities', of whom the lesbian and gay communities are the most vocal, organized and challenging (Wilson 1995; Rayside 1998). The idea of sexual citizenship has many features in common with other claims to citizenship. It is about enfranchisement, about inclusion, about belonging, about equity and justice, about rights balanced by new responsibilities. What is different about it is that it is bringing to the fore issues and struggles that were only implicit or silenced in earlier notions of citizenship. On one level, as already suggested, these are old issues newly rearticulated in the concept of sexual citizenship. But the idea of sexual citizenship goes much further than this. It is an attempt to put on the agenda issues that have only fully come to the fore since the 1960s, and have now moved from the margins to the centre of our concerns because of very powerful cultural and social changes (see, for examples, the essays in Weeks and Holland 1996).

Conclusion

I have offered a general analysis of what I am calling an unfinished revolution. It is a revolution without a set goal, or a clear path. It is an odd mixture of long term trends and everyday experiments. Many will argue that when we look at the victims of these changes, whether children, abandoned mothers, single mothers living in poverty, sexually transmitted diseases and the like, the changes may not be worth the candle. But I am suggesting that amidst all the admitted casualties of change, there are many gains: in the emergence of new balances between autonomy and mutuality, in greater toleration of diversity, and in a broadening concept of what it is to belong, to be a full citizen. I chose as my title a play on an old phrase, that was supposed to characterize the British way: 'live and let live' – a type of toleration which was based on indifference, rather than acceptance. I also couldn't help remembering the old James Bond title, 'live and let die', which certainly is apt for some of our sexual history. I wanted to suggest that we are moving into a more positive era, not just accepting the fact of diversity, but embracing diversity as a strong norm to be achieved, which is what I wanted to suggest with 'live and let love' – hopefully, one day, without the question mark I give it, for the time being, in my title.

References

Adam, B.D. (1992) 'Sex and Caring among Men: Impacts of AIDS on Gay People', in K. Plummer (ed.) *Modern Homosexualities: Fragments of Lesbian and Gay Experience*, London: Routledge: 175–83.

Andrews, G. (ed.) (1991) *Citizenship*, London: Lawrence and Wishart.

Anthias, F. and Yuval-Davis, N. (1992) *Racialized Boundaries: Race, Nation, Gender, Colour and Class, and the Anti-racist Struggle*, London: Routledge.

Beck, U. and Beck-Gernsheim, E. (1995) *The Normal Chaos of Love*, Cambridge: Polity Press.

Bell, D. and Binnie, J. (2000) *The Sexual Citizen*, Cambridge: Polity Press

Bhatt, C. (1997) *Liberation and Purity: Race, New Religious Movements and the Ethics of Postmodernity*, London: UCL Press.

Bhabha, H. (1990) 'The Third Space', in J. Rutherford (ed.) *Identity: Community, Culture, Difference*, London: Lawrence and Wishart.

Blasius, M. (1994) *Gay and Lesbian Politics: Sexuality and the Emergence of a New Ethic*, Philadelphia: Temple University Press.

Boyes, R. (2000) 'Sterilisation law reveals Sweden's repressive state', *The Times*, 31 March, p. 19.

Butler, J. (1990) *Gender Trouble: Feminism and the Subversion of Identity*, New York and London: Routledge.

Cooper, D. (1995) *Power in Struggle: Feminism, Sexuality and the State*, Buckingham: Open University Press.

Donovan, C., Heaphy, B. and Weeks, J. (2000) 'Citizenship and Same Sex Relationships', *Journal of Social Policy* 28(4): 689–709.

Duggan, L. and Hunter, N.D. (1995) *Sex Wars: Sexual Dissent and Political Culture*, New York and London: Routledge.

Durkheim, E. (1974) *Sociology and Philosophy*, New York: The Free Press.

Durham, M. (1997) 'Conservative Agendas and Government Policy', in L. Segal (1997): 90–100.

Dunne, G. (1997) *Lesbian Lifestyles: Women's Work and the Politics of Sexuality*, Basingstoke and London: Macmillan.

Epstein, D., Johnson, R. and Steinberg, D.L. (2000) 'Twice Told Tales: Transformation, Recuperation and Emergence in the Age of Consent Debates 1998', *Sexualities* 3(1), February: 5–30.

Epstein, S. (1996) *Pure Science: AIDS, Activism, and the Politics of Knowledge*, Berkeley, Los Angeles and London: University of California Press.

Etzioni, A. (1995) *The Spirit of Community: Rights, Responsibilities and the Communitarian Agenda*, London: Fontana Press.

Evans, D. (1993) *Sexual Citizenship: The Material Construction of Sexualities*, London: Routledge.

—— (1995) '(Homo)sexual Citizenship: A Queer Kind of Justice', in A.R. Wilson (ed.) (1995).

Feminist Review (1997) 'Citizenship: Pushing the Boundaries'. 57, Autumn.

Finch, J. and Mason, J. (1993) *Negotiating Family Responsibilities*, London: Routledge.

Foucault, M. (1979) *The History of Sexuality, Volume 1. An Introduction*. London: Allen Lane.

Foucault, M. (1988) 'The ethic of care for the self as a practice of freedom', in J. Bernauer and D. Rasmussen (eds) *The Final Foucault*, Cambridge, Ma.: The MIT Press.

Fukuyama, F. (1999) *The Great Disruption: Human Nature and the Reconstitution of Social Order*, London: Profile Books.

Gagnon, J. and Simon, W. (1974) *Sexual Conduct: The Social Sources of Human Sexuality*, London: Hutchinson.

Garber, M. (1992) *Vested Interests: Cross-Dressing and Cultural Anxiety*, New York and London: Routledge.

Giddens, A. (1990) *The Consequences of Modernity*, Cambridge: Polity Press.

—— (1991) *Modernity and Self Identity: Self and Society in the late Modern Age*, Cambridge: Polity Press.

—— (1992) *The Transformation of Intimacy: Sexuality, Love and Eroticism in Modern Societies*, Cambridge: Polity Press.

—— (1994) *Beyond Left and Right: The Future of Radical Politics*, Cambridge: Polity Press.

Heller, A. (1984) *Everyday Life*, London: Routledge and Kegan Paul.

Herman, D. (1997) *The Antigay Agenda: Orthodox Vision and the Christian Right*, Chicago and London: Chicago University Press.

Holland, J., Ramazanoglu, C., Sharpe, S. and Thomson, R. (1998) *The Male in the Head: Young People, Heterosexuality and Power*, London: The Tufnell Press.

Jamieson, L. (1998) *Intimacy: Personal Relationships in Modern Societies*, Cambridge: Polity Press.

Kaplan, M.B. (1997) *Sexual Justice: Democratic Citizenship and the Politics of Desire*, New York and London: Routledge.

Lister, R. (1996) 'Citizenship Engendered', in D. Taylor (ed.) *Critical Social Policy: A Reader*, London: Sage.

Lister, R. (1997) *Citizenship: Feminist Perspectives*, Basingstoke and London: Macmillan.

Marshall, T.H. (1950) *Citizenship and Social Class*, Cambridge: Cambridge University Press.

Melucci, A. (1996) *The Playing Self: Person and Meaning in the Planetary Society*, Cambridge: Cambridge University Press.

Mort, F. (1987) *Dangerous Sexualities: Medico-Moral Politics in England Since 1830*, London: Routledge and Kegan Paul.

Mulgan, G. (1997) *Connexity: How to Live in a Connected World*, London: Chatto and Windus.

Plummer, K. (1995) *Telling Sexual Stories: Power, Change, and Social Worlds*, London: Routledge.

Rayside, D. (1998) *On the Fringe: Gays and Lesbians in the Political Process*, Ithaca and London: Cornell University Press.

Richardson, D. (1998) 'Sexuality and Citizenship', *Sociology* 32(1): 83–100.

Segal, L. (ed.) (1997) *New Sexual Agendas*, Basingstoke and London: Macmillan.

Sinfield, A. (1997) 'Queer Identities and the Ethnicity Model', in Segal (1997): 196–204.

Sullivan, A. (ed.) (1997) *Same-Sex Marriage: Pro and Con: A Reader*, New York: Vintage Books.

Turner, B. (ed.) (1993) *Citizenship and Social Theory*. London: Sage.

Walby, S. (1994) 'Is Citizenship Gendered?' *Sociology* 28(1): 379–95.

Watney, S. (1994) *Practices of Freedom: Selected Writings on HIV/AIDS*. London: Rivers Oram Press.

Weeks, J. (1981/1989) *Sex, Politics and Social Change: The Regulation of Sexuality since 1800*, Harlow: Longman.

—— (1985) *Sexuality and its Discontents: Meanings, Myths and Modern Sexualities*, London: Routledge.

—— (1995) *Invented Moralities: Sexual Values in an Age of Uncertainty*, Cambridge: Polity Press.

—— (1998) 'The Sexual Citizen', *Theory, Culture and Society* 15(3–4): 35–52.

—— (2000) *Making Sexual History*, Cambridge: Polity Press.

Weeks, J., Donovan, C. and Heaphy, B. (1998) 'Everyday Experiments: Narratives of Non-Heterosexual Relationships', in E. Silva and C. Smart (eds), *The New Family?* London: Sage.

—— (1999) 'Families of Choice: Autonomy and Mutuality in Non-heterosexual Relationships', in S. McRae (ed.) *Changing Britain: Population and Household Change*, Oxford: Oxford University Press.

Weeks, J. and Holland, J. (eds) (1996) *Sexual Cultures: Communities, Values and Intimacy*, Basingstoke and London: Macmillan.

Wellings, K., Field, J., Johnson, A. and Wadsworth, J. (1994) *Sexual Behaviour in Britain: The National Survey of Sexual Attitudes and Lifestyles*, London: Penguin.

Weston, K. (1991) *Families We Choose*, New York: Columbia University Press.

Wilson, A.R. (ed.) (1995) *A Simple Matter of Justice? Theorizing Lesbian and Gay Politics*, London: Cassell.

Wolmark, J. (ed.) (1999) *Cybersexualities: A Reader in Feminist Theory, Cyborgs and Cyberspace*, Edinburgh: Edinburgh University Press.

Woodhead, D. (1998) *Safer Sexual Citizenship: The Effects of Community Development Sexual Health Promotion on HIV negative Gay Men in the AIDS epidemic*, unpublished Ph.D. thesis, South Bank University, London.

Chapter 5

Widening the scope of social policy

Families, financial services and the impact of technology

Jan Pahl

Social policy analysts have traditionally been concerned with the financial welfare provided by the state in the form of social security payments, means tested benefits and tax allowances. However, the past twenty years have seen a dramatic expansion in the financial services provided by the private sector, which now involves seven per cent of the GDP and employs more people than the National Health Service (Treasury Committee 1999b: 69). So should the scope of social policy be extended to include the financial services sector and its impact on financial welfare?

Being a full citizen of Western European society increasingly depends on access to financial products and services, that is access to credit, banking facilities, mortgages, insurance and so on. However, the reality is that one and a half million households lack even the most basic of financial products, such as a current bank account and home contents insurance, while a further 4.4 million are on the margins of financial exclusion, using just one or two financial products (Kempson and Whyley 1999).

One response might be to say that financial services are located in the private sector, and as such are outside the scope of social policy, which has traditionally been concerned with the public sector. However, over the past twenty years the role of the state in the provision of welfare has changed from that of provider to one in which providing, purchasing and regulating are all significant in determining the welfare of individuals and families. The regulatory state is increasingly of concern to social policy analysts.

The relevance of this point was underlined by the evidence which Patricia Hewitt, MP and at that time Economic Secretary to the Treasury, presented to the Treasury Select Committee when it considered the proposals for the Financial Services and Markets Bill and the arrangements for the new Financial Services Authority. Hewitt commented, 'Financial markets, well run and well regulated, are vital to individuals' and families' security' (Treasury Committee 1999b: 69).

The aim of this chapter is to consider the implications for social policy of changes in the use of financial services, and particularly the use of credit cards and banking, in the light of recent research on family financial arrangements and new forms of money (Pahl 1999). The research was the first to examine the ways in which the complex world of personal and family finances is adapting to the electronic economy. Are new forms of money constraining or enhancing the access which individuals have to the money which enters the household in which they are living? If access to financial services is becoming part of citizenship, are some people more fully citizens than others?

The research developed out of a long-standing interest in the control and allocation of money within the family (Pahl 1989). This work has shown that couples manage their finances in a great variety of different ways. Some couples pool all their income, typically in a joint bank account, and attach considerable importance to financial equality. Other couples maintain independence in financial matters, dividing responsibility for the payment of joint bills and attaching importance to privacy and autonomy in financial matters.

Some couples give overall financial control to one partner or the other, while others divide finances into separate spheres, making each partner responsible for specific areas of spending. The most recent evidence, from the British Household Panel Survey, suggests that about half of all couples pool their incomes and share management of the pool. In about a third of couples finances are managed by the wife, while in about one sixth they are managed by the husband, typically with a housekeeping allowance being transferred to the wife. Finally, a small but growing number of couples hold and manage their money as though they were still two separate individuals. (See for example, Brannen and Wilson 1987; Burgoyne and Morison 1997; Buck *et al*. 1994; Goode, Callender and Lister 1998; Laurie 1996; Morris and Ruane 1989; Nyman 1999; Pahl 1989, 1995; Vogler and Pahl 1993, 1994; Wilson 1987).

New forms of money and the growth of the electronic economy

Most previous research on family finances essentially conceptualized money as cash, or as cash held in a bank account. However, over the past thirty years there have been profound changes in the ways in which ordinary people receive, hold and spend their money. The first credit card was launched in 1966, to be followed by store cards, debit cards, loyalty cards and smart or chargeable cards (Credit Card Research Group, 1998). Banking by telephone or computer began in the 1980s, with an accelerating expansion in the use of electronic banking services throughout the 1990s. All these developments are described here as 'new forms of money' or as the 'electronic economy'.

The mix of non-cash payments varies greatly between countries, with two extremes being represented by the United States and Sweden (Cruickshank 2000: 61). In 1997 the United States still relied heavily on cheques, which made up 74 per cent of all non-cash payments, compared with 2 per cent in Sweden. By contrast credit transfers made up 73 per cent of non-cash transfers in Sweden, compared with 2 per cent in the United States. Credit card payments made up 19 per cent of all non-cash transfers in the United States, compared with just 1 per cent in Sweden. The United Kingdom had a more evenly balanced pattern of payments, with 31 per cent of transactions being carried out by cheque, 19 per cent by credit transfer, 13 per cent by credit card and 18 per cent by debit card. From the point of the providers of financial services, cash and cheques are the most expensive forms of payment and credit transfers the cheapest, while credit card payments are rather more expensive to process than payments by debit card. This leads to service providers giving privileges to those who use the cheaper forms of payment and penalizing those who continue to use the more expensive methods, such as cash and cheques.

Telephone and internet banking are creating turmoil in what was once a sedate and secure industry. Again the penetration varies greatly between different countries. Banks in the UK have been very successful in promoting the use of telephone banking, so that around 10 per cent of customers banked by phone in 1997/98, a rate higher than that of any other European country except France. However, the pattern for internet banking was rather different, with the UK lagging behind the Scandinavian countries. One review found that around 5 per cent of UK current account holders were either using or had a very strong interest in using PC/internet banking. The use of internet banking was disproportionately weighted in favour of younger customers (particularly those aged 21 to 34 years), those of higher social class and those with higher earnings (Cruickshank 2000: 29).

Methods of the study

Money is a sensitive and private subject. All researchers know that asking people about their finances can be more intrusive than asking about sexual relations. In addition, this study was essentially exploratory. Therefore it seemed important to use a variety of research methods, partly in order to throw the investigative net as widely as possible, and partly to gain experience about the acceptability and validity of different methods, in a way which might benefit future research on the topic.

Three different sources of data were used, in order to gain both quantitative and qualitative information about the issues which were being explored. First, analyses of the 1993/94 Family Expenditure Survey (FES) provided quantitative data about 3676 married couples, which could be generalized to a larger population because of the nature of the survey. The FES collects information about the income and expenditure of the household, and in addition each individual spender is asked to complete an expenditure diary, listing every item bought over a period of two weeks and noting whether a credit card was used to make the purchase (Office of National Statistics 1996).

Second, seven focus groups took place, involving 59 individuals living in five different parts of England. Finally, face-to-face interviews were carried out with 40 couples, in order to develop a more qualitative understanding of the ways in which individuals and couples managed their finances and made use of new forms of money. Men and women were interviewed separately and privately.

Cluster analysis of credit card use

As an introduction to the issues with which this paper is concerned, we begin by examining the use of credit cards, drawing on quantitative data from the FES and qualitative data from three interviews. Explorations of the FES data had suggested that the use of credit cards was statistically associated with a number of different variables, among which income, employment status and age at the end of full time education were particularly important. Clearly such variables were interrelated in a complex way. A statistical cluster analysis was used to create a new classification of individuals which would examine the relationships between these variables. The aim was to identify clusters of individuals with common characteristics and to investigate patterns of credit card use for each cluster. Further information about the statistical techniques used for the cluster analysis and about the characteristics of the individuals in each cluster is given in Pahl (1999).

In order to examine the interlocking effects of the different variables, the statistical computer package was asked to define six clusters, basing the clusters on age at the end of full time education, the income of each partner and the employment status of the couple. The cluster analysis was carried out separately for men and women, so the totals in each cluster are not exactly the same for each sex.

Cluster 1 contained a high proportion of individuals who were retired or living in households with no paid work. The majority of both men and women in this cluster had ended their education at 14 or 15 and incomes were uniformly low. For most of the households in this cluster, social class was not recorded in the FES. So a typical member of cluster 1 had left school at the minimum age and was *unemployed or retired*.

Cluster 2 contained many couples where the woman was either in part time employment or did not have a job. In this cluster women's incomes were substantially lower than those of the men, despite their similar levels of education Typically the head of the household was classified as being a skilled manual worker, though this cluster also contained some retired people. So the typical couple in cluster 2 was a *skilled manual worker whose wife had part time or no paid work.*

Cluster 3 contained many couples in which both partners were in full time employment, with the relatively low income levels of the men being balanced by the relatively high incomes of the women. This suggested that these were couples where having two earners was necessary in order to make ends meet. The women tended to have had more years of education than the men. In terms of social class, these were households where the 'head' was likely to come from social class II or be a skilled manual worker. This combination of characteristics suggests that cluster 3 might be described as *middle income, dual job couples*.

Cluster 4 contained many households where the man had a full-time job, while the woman had no paid work or only a part time job. This cluster was characterized by medium levels of education for both men and women. However, there was a substantial gender gap in terms of income, with men typically earning much more than women. In terms of social class, the 'head of household' was likely to be classified as social class I or II. So a typical couple in cluster 4 might be characterized as *middle-class, with a breadwinner husband and a home maker wife.*

Cluster 5 was a cluster in which most women were in full- or part-time employment, and in which many were the main earners for the households in which they lived. Typically it contained individuals who had relatively low educational levels, with most people leaving school at 15 or 16. Among men, especially, their low educational levels were translated into relatively low incomes, with most 'heads of household' being classified as social class IIIM. By contrast women's incomes were at medium levels for women in the sample, suggesting that many had jobs classified as social class III, non-manual. So cluster 5 could be described as the *low income, dual job couples.*

Cluster 6 contained the most highly educated individuals in the sample, with both men and women typically having completed some years of higher education. The effect of this showed in the relatively high income levels for both men and women, and in a social class classification which placed the majority in social classes I and II, with both partners being in full-time employment. Typically these were *high income, dual career couples with professional jobs.*

The cluster analysis inevitably simplified the complexity of reality. However, it did make it possible to group households according to some key structural variables. As we shall see, the variations between clusters were reflected in very significant differences in the use of credit cards.

Use of credit cards by clusters of households

Table 5.1 gives the percentages of individuals in each cluster who had used a credit card during the two weeks during which the expenditure diaries were being kept. The most striking variations were between the different clusters: these were highly significant for both women and men. Thus, at one extreme, 68 per cent of men in cluster 6 had used a credit card to make a purchase, while, at the other extreme, only 8 per cent of women in cluster 1 had used a credit card during the two weeks when the survey took place. As we have seen, cluster 6 contained the most highly educated and best paid couples in the sample, while cluster 1 was predominantly composed of people who were retired or unemployed.

Credit card use was highest in cluster 6, for both men and women, but it was also relatively high among men in cluster 4. These were the middle-class couples in which the men were typically the sole or the main earners. Their status as breadwinners may have given these men more confidence in money matters, while the women's lack of an independent income may have made it harder for them to get a credit card in their own right, and discouraged them from spending money which they had not earned themselves on the relatively expensive goods which are typically bought with credit cards. A similar pattern existed in cluster 2, which contained a majority of couples in which the man was in full-time employment,

Table 5.1 Six clusters by percentages of women and men using a credit card to make a purchase over a two week period

| | Cluster number | | | | | |
	1	2	3	4	5	6
Percentage of women who used a credit card	8	20	40	42	23	63
Total number	965	916	332	515	659	289
$p < 0.0001$						
Percentage of men who used a credit card	11	24	33	52	22	68
Total number	979	872	298	533	713	281

$p < 0.0001$

while the woman was in part-time work, or did not have a paid job. The lower overall use of credit cards in cluster 2 reflects the fact that most of the men were in manual occupations, while cluster 4 contained a majority of men in non-manual occupations.

There were two clusters in which women were more likely than men to have made use of a credit card. The first was cluster 3, in which 40 per cent of women had used a credit card, compared with 33 per cent of men. This was the cluster in which women tended to be better paid and better educated than the men, and this finding underlined yet again the importance of income and education in explaining credit card use.

The second cluster in which marginally more women than men used a credit card was cluster 5, which, as we have seen, contained the largest number of couples in which women were the main earners. This was also the cluster in which both partners were likely to be in full-time employment, with most of the men in jobs classified as skilled working class. Evidence from the focus groups suggested that this was a group in which many women felt confident with new forms of money, in a way which the men did not.

Perhaps the most striking finding to come from the cluster analysis was the importance of education. Making comparisons between the different clusters underlined the extent to which credit card use reflected, not simply personal tastes and choices, but the economic context within which individuals and couples lived their lives. It might be expected that the use of credit cards would reflect economic variables such as income and employment, but it was surprising to see the importance of age at the end of full-time education.

In order to illuminate the reality which lies behind these figures we turn next to three case studies from the interviews, selected in order to reflect three of the ideal types which were identified by the cluster analysis.

A dual career couple using many new forms of money

Cluster 6 drew together a group of well educated individuals, in full-time jobs, whose incomes were relatively high by comparison with the rest of the sample, and who were classified as belonging to social classes I or II. Around two thirds of both men and women in this cluster had used a credit card during the two weeks of the FES survey.

Andrea and Michael were typical of cluster 6. Aged in their twenties, they both had degrees. They had no children and their full-time jobs as a tax consultant and a teacher gave them a joint income of just under £50,000 gross per year, or over £600 per week net. When shown a list of different financial arrangements and asked to pick the one which came closest to their own, both picked the system described as 'We pool some of our money and keep some of it separately'. As Andrea said,

> We put an amount in every month from each of our personal accounts into the joint account. Then from the joint account goes all the joint expenditure, like mortgage, bills, etc., etc. Then what is left in our own personal account is for our own use.

They had a credit card on the joint account in Andrea's name, for joint expenditure, and a number of other credit and debit cards for personal use. They used these cards for almost all their shopping and monitored spending carefully, paying the bills in full every month and never paying any interest. Michael described how this worked in practice:

> If it's a joint thing then we'd put it on her Barclaycard, and if it was business, it obviously comes off my business account, and if it's for going home to my parents, then I pay – that comes out of my money – and if we're going to her parents, then it comes out of her money. Presents? We each look after our own families.

Michael had a gold card and his comments underlined the symbolic significance of some new forms of money:

> Depending on who I'm with, if I want to vaguely impress them, I'll get out the gold card. If they get out their gold card, and we're splitting the meal fifty/fifty, then I whack mine on the table and that, er, gives some kind of credibility I suppose.

Neither used much cash and both were scathing about loyalty cards. They had thought about telephone and computer banking, but for the time being were satisfied with their existing arrangements. Their system enabled them to save and Michael was building up a portfolio of shares.

Previous research on money and marriage has developed typologies to describe the different ways in which couples control their finances (see, for example, Pahl 1989; Vogler and Pahl 1993). Andrea and Michael were using 'partial pooling', a system characteristic of couples where both are earning. Their careful balancing of joint and separate spending represented the tension between their joint lives together and the expectations of their separate families of origin. Having enough money enabled them to use new forms of money to manage their finances and, on occasion, to impress others. Their situation was very different from that of the couples in cluster 1.

An unemployed couple with credit card debts

Cluster 1 in Table 5.1 drew together a group of individuals who were typically dependent on state benefits, either because they were retired or because they were unemployed. Tom and Teresa, aged 25, unemployed and with two young children, were finding it hard to make ends meet. Tom's Job Seeker's Allowance was paid into his bank account, while the payments for Income Support, Child Benefit and Housing Benefit were paid into Teresa's bank account. He gave her money towards the bills, but also liked to have something left to spend on hi fi equipment.

When asked about their financial arrangements, Tom and Teresa chose the option, 'We pool all our money and manage our household finances jointly', but in the separate interviews both said that Teresa was really responsible for making ends meet: when family income is low women tend to get the job of making ends meet. He said, 'I leave it all up to her'. She said,

I have to remind him that there's things to pay and that he can't just go out and squander money. I get very worried about money, you see. If I haven't paid something I won't sleep. I have to pay my bills. And whatever I've got left I'll live on it. I can live on like a fiver a week, if I have to. But he says things like, 'We only live once'. You know, 'You're always going to get money'. But I think you have to pay bills to survive.

Tom explained his attitude in terms of his family of origin:

I'm not really money oriented. The family that I've been with hasn't really been money oriented. Whereas she, Teresa, should I say, she's from that different area and class. So she's got more responsibility with money than what I have. I'm quite glad she's there, because if she wasn't there, I'd spend all me money.

Their current financial problems were exacerbated by the fact that when she had been in work they had used her Visa card to pay for a holiday. They had taken out money up to and above her credit limit and were still paying off what they owed. She complained,

> I think it's ridiculous. I don't think you should have to pay interest on any cards or your accounts. They get enough money out of you as it is. I mean I've only got £500 over the limit and some people have got thousands and thousands on it.

> Q. *What do you feel when you're using your credit card?*

> I don't really know I'm doing it. Like I say, it's a piece of plastic and it's not like handing cash over. No, it's plastic money. It's lies. You don't feel you're spending anything.

The interviewer asked Tom whether he was thinking of getting a new card:

> Um . . . yes and no. 'Yes' because the simple fact is, like I say, it's as good as money, and you've got it on you whenever you need it. 'No' because there's sometimes you can overspend money, without knowing.

> Q. *What did you feel when you had a card and you used it?*

> I thought, 'Yeah, I've got this credit card here, and now I can go buy what I want, when I want'. Because I know, if I want something, that I will definitely get it. Most definitely.

Teresa and Tom were operating the system of financial management which in previous research has been described as 'wife management' or the 'whole wage system'. This system is characteristic of low income families. As in this example, the man's lack of involvement in financial matters can serve to protect his personal spending money and keep off the agenda the woman's struggles to make ends meet (Vogler 1998). For this couple, and especially for Tom, new forms of money, such as credit cards, offer an opportunity for personal spending which can undermine the woman's struggle to make ends meet for the household as a whole.

A breadwinner husband who controlled finances

A contrasting picture was presented by those couples who fell into Cluster 4 in Table 1, which was typified by a middle-class, breadwinner husband with a wife who had no paid work or just a part-time job. Derek and Helen were in this category. He had left school at 18 and was an estate agent, while she had left school at 16 and now worked part time in an office. They had three teenage children. There was a great disparity in their salaries, since she earned under £10,000, while he received at least £42,000 per annum gross, and may have earned much more, since this was the top point on the salary scale from which respondents were invited to identify how much they earned.

Both saw him as the main earner and both considered that he controlled the family finances. They had a joint account, into which his salary was paid, while her salary was paid into her own account. She described how their system worked, and it was clear that, like many women in her situation, she did not feel comfortable about spending 'his' money:

> We have a joint account into which his money goes and the household expenditure is made from. So I'm very strict with myself about what I spend money from that account on. It won't be on things for me, because I have my own account for that. And it gives me a sense of independence to be able to do that.

Derek confirmed what she had said,

> I mean, basically, I provide the money. She has her own independence now, but most of the money that comes into the household is mine. And the money that Helen earns, I don't touch at all. Dare I say absolute pin money or whatever. It's a bit of a chauvinistic statement that, but I'm not ashamed.

They have a joint Visa card, which is paid out of their joint account, and a joint debit card, and she has several store cards, which she pays from her own account. He also has an American Express card. In the past she had had her own Barclaycard, but Derek had disapproved of the fact that she was paying high interest rates on her outstanding balance. She described what happened:

> Derek said to me, 'Look, you're paying through the nose on your Barclaycard – really high interest rates. I'm going to get you transferred to the Cooperative Bank'. Well I wasn't too keen, to be honest with you, because my Barclaycard I'd had since I was at work. So it was my sort of account, in my name. I didn't want to be second named on his account. Silly sort of thing really. So I sort of kicked my heels over this one for a little bit, cutting my nose to spite my face, and in the end sort of gave in. So now Derek gets the statements on our joint Visa card. Which in a way I don't really like, because he knows now what I'm spending with my credit card. I like to have some sort of mysteries in my life.

Her husband, in his own separate interview, described the same incident, but threw rather a different light on it:

> Helen was Barclaycard and she had about £1500 on there. She was being charged 17 or 18 per cent, which is dire. They were offering a freebie at the Coop, so I applied for a card, got her balance transferred over and they paid off the Barclaycard. Cut that up, and got rid of it at a special incentive rate of six per cent for the first six months. I paid some of it for her, but I didn't pay the whole lot off, because – perhaps it's my thing – I've never discussed it

> with her as a discipline thing, that yes, I could pay it off, because I bring the money in. But it's important for Helen to contribute towards it, because she spent the money, you see.

The story of her credit card reflects a more general situation in which he ultimately controlled finances. When asked about making a major purchasing decision, she said,

> We would discuss it. But I would have to say, ultimately the decision would lie with Derek. And I think that boils down to the fact that he earns the money. It's as simple as that.

Derek and Helen were operating the system of financial management described in previous research as 'male controlled pooling', but with a strong ideology of the male as breadwinner, which is reflected in his control of finances and Helen's feeling that she has no right to spend 'his' money on herself. The dispute about her credit card illustrated his power to control the discussion (Vogler 1998). This couple underlined the point that two individuals living in the same household can have access to different amounts of money, can vary in their right to spend that money, and can have different standards of living. They may also keep secrets from each other.

The patterns which emerged from the research were complex, but they suggested an increasing polarization in terms of access to the electronic economy. Those who were making full use of new forms of money tended to be 'work rich', in that they belonged to households with more than one earner, 'credit rich', in that their credit rating was secure, and 'information rich', in that they felt confident of their ability to manipulate the financial market place for their own advantage.

At the other extreme, some individuals were more or less excluded from the electronic economy. They tended to be 'work poor', typically living in households without a regular earner, 'credit poor', in that it was hard for them to get any sort of loan, and 'information poor', in that they did not understand the rules of the new world of personal finance.

Within marriage new forms of money seemed to be altering the balance between 'our' money and 'my' money, allowing 'credit rich' individuals to pursue their own financial goals without consulting their partners, and generally increasing the difference in power between those who earn and those who are dependent on them. This is a complex area which is being explored very fruitfully by Singh (1997, see also Singh and Ryan, 1999).

Patterns of financial exclusion

The results of this study can be set in a broader context by looking at the growing literature on financial exclusion, defined as having few or no financial products. Important work on this topic is being done at the Personal Finance Research Centre at the University of Bristol. A regression analysis of data from the Family Resources Survey identified the factors which were most significant in predicting financial exclusion. These were:

- being in receipt of means tested benefits
- having a low household income
- having been out of work for some time
- renting a home
- being a single person, non-pensioner household
- belonging to the Pakistani or Bangladeshi communities
- having left school before the age of 16
- living in Scotland or in one of the 50 most deprived local authorities in England and Wales.

Financial exclusion has been shown to be a complex and dynamic process (Kempson and Whyley 1999). Some people have spent all their lives in a cash-based economy, with pensioners and the long-term unemployed being over-represented among this group. Others have given up using financial services, often because of a drop in income following unemployment or retirement. Women may cease to use financial services on the death of a partner in whose name the products were held. The majority of people without financial products are excluded by a combination of marketing, pricing and inappropriate product design. However, a small group has either been refused access to financial products or has made a conscious decision not to use them (Kempson and Whyley 1999; see also Ford 1991; Lewis *et al*. 1997; Molloy and Snape 1999).

Changes in the world of banking will affect patterns of social exclusion in the future. In 1988 National Westminster bank, Barclays Bank and Midland Bank (now HSBC) had between them 7,888 branches; by 1999 this figure had been reduced to 5,233 (Ibison 2000: 3). A report by Deloitte Consultancy estimated that one third of bank branches will close by the year 2004 (Brown-Humes 1999). Branches in the poorer parts of cities and in rural areas are especially likely to be affected by this process of retrenchment, which reflects the unprofitability of small accounts and of low-income customers. The recent closure of 172 branch banks was defended by Barclays, on the grounds that the bank had 1.2 million telephone banking customers and 650,000 on line customers (Ibison, Newman and Tighe 2000: 3)

Changes in technology mean that the current generation of credit and debit cards will be replaced by smart cards. These contain a silicon chip processor with a memory. Smart cards can do all that debit and credit cards can do, but can also hold money in different currencies and store information such as passport and identity details, supermarket loyalty points and health records (Brown-Humes 1998a). In the future smart cards will be linked to computer operating systems, making it possible to access electronic cash and on-line shopping from the home computer (Cole 1999: 12). However, some research has suggested that, compared with men, women are less at home with, and less likely to use the new technologies associated with financial products (Singh and Ryan 1999).

Policy debates about financial services and new technologies

The financial lives of individuals are located on the crossroads between the state and the market, between the public and the private sectors. On the one hand, the state regulates the financial situation of every citizen, through the tax system, the social security system and a myriad other controls on wages, salaries, interest rates and prices. On the other hand, the financial services sector epitomizes the free flowing nature of market capitalism in a global economy; any interference by policy makers is likely to be seen as threatening the efficient working of the system. In this context, making proposals for policy may be a dangerous enterprise. However, it is clear that social policy analysts cannot any longer ignore the implications of changes in financial services and in the information technology which gives access to those services (Cahill 1994). In the space available here it is only possible to mention three policy areas.

First, access to financial education and unbiased information about financial services is likely to be increasingly important. Shortly after taking office, the Labour government announced a new system for the regulation of financial services, and in 1997 concentrated powers in a new body, called the Financial Services Authority. This is responsible for informing the public about the financial products that are available, encouraging the development of more flexible products and ensuring that relevant information is available for consumers (Treasury Committee 1999a; see also the Financial Services Authority 1998). The government also initiated the Financial Services and Markets Bill, which at the time of writing was passing through Parliament. There has been some concern about the extent to which financial advice and education are available to those who need them most (National Consumer Council 1999). Those who are less likely to use financial services tend to be those for whom accessing education and advice are also difficult. It has also been suggested that the design and marketing of many financial products reflects masculine conceptions of time and traditional male patterns of employment (Knight and Odih 1995).

Second, there is the issue of financial exclusion and access to banking and credit. The minutes of the Treasury Select Committee, which considered the new provisions for financial regulation, made it clear that financial exclusion was expected to be of concern to the Financial Services Authority. Patricia Hewitt MP, Economic Secretary to the Treasury, giving evidence to the Select Committee, said,

> We want to see a financial services industry in this country that is offering all consumers or potential consumers the advice, where that is appropriate, and the product that they need to meet their particular needs.
>
> (Treasury Committee 1999b: 79)

She expressed concern about the difficulties faced by individuals without bank accounts and communities without branch banks, and went on to mention the task force on credit unions and banks which has been established within the Treasury.

In a consumer society access to credit is becoming an important aspect of welfare. Credit allows individuals to smooth out the peaks and troughs in their incomes and to purchase those goods and services which they require, even though they do not currently have enough money. However, it is clear that some individuals and some households are excluded from the mainstream credit-based society; if they do use credit it tends to be from more expensive sources (Kempson 1994; Rowlingson 1994; Rowlingson and Kempson 1994). In a consumer society, the poor too easily become defined as 'flawed consumers', to use the phrase coined by Bauman (1998).

This is the context for the current revival of interest in credit unions. A credit union is 'a cooperative society offering its members loans out of the pool of savings built up by the members themselves' (Berthoud and Hinton 1989: 1, see also Conaty and Mayo 1997). The aim is to provide accessible credit at reasonable rates of interest to groups based on a locality or a workplace, and to give people a sense of taking control over their finances. Britain has a much less well-developed system of credit unions than some other countries, despite attempts by local authorities to encourage them. This is largely because of the restrictions imposed by the 1979 Credit Unions Act, which prevents credit unions from giving unsecured loans for more than two years, caps loans at £5000 above what a member has saved and limits membership to a maximum of 5,000 people (Berthoud and Hinton, 1989; Leyshon, Thrift and Justice, 1993). Changes which have been proposed include lifting the present limit on the numbers of members, extending the loan repayment period and allowing credit unions to offer other financial services (Brown-Humes 1998b).

Access to banking facilities is likely to become increasingly important, especially in the light of pressure to pay social security benefits into bank accounts. In the USA the Community Reinvestment Act imposes an obligation on banks to endeavour to meet the credit needs of their local communities (Oppenheim 1998: 177). The British government is clearly concerned about this issue, with Melanie Johnson, Economic Secretary to the Treasury, announcing as this chapter is being written that the government expects all the main banks to be running basic accounts for low income groups by October 2000 (*Financial Times*, 13 April 2000: 4).

Third, the control and allocation of money within the family continues to be an issue. New forms of money seem to be individualizing family finances and making it easier for higher earners to spend without consulting their partners and to control the spending of those who are financially dependent upon them. Men tend to make more use of new technologies than women do, and this difference is being translated into a greater use of telephone and internet banking (Singh and Ryan 1999). So within marriage new forms of money may be altering the balance between 'our' money and 'my' money in a way which has profound implications for social policy. The household is the basic unit for many decisions about access to financial products and services, but citizenship is essentially an attribute of an individual and not of the household in which s/he lives.

Acknowledgements

This research was funded by the Joseph Rowntree Foundation and the University of Kent at Canterbury: I am pleased to have this opportunity to thank both for their support. I am also grateful to all those who worked on the project, and especially the members of the Advisory Group, who were immensely helpful and generous. Professor Lou Opit worked on the analyses of the FES until four days before his death in May 1998: this chapter is dedicated to him with my love.

References

Bauman, Z. (1998) *Work, Consumerism and the New Poor*, Buckingham: Open University Press

Berthoud, R. and Hinton, T. (1989) *Credit Unions in the United Kingdom*, London: Policy Studies Institute.

Brannen, J., and Wilson, G. (1987) *Give and Take in Families: Studies in Resource Distribution*, London: Allen and Unwin.

Brown-Humes, C. (1998a) 'Where smart money is headed', *Financial Times*, 11 July.

—— (1998b) 'Banking in the aisles', *Financial Times*, 16 May.

—— (1999) 'Technological advance drives revolution', *Financial Times*, 7 July.

Buck, N., Gershuny, J., Rose, D. and Scott, J. (1994) *Changing Households: the British Household Panel Survey 1990–1992*, Colchester: University of Essex.

Burgoyne, C. and Morison, V. (1997) 'Money in re-marriage: keeping things separate – but simple', *Sociological Review* 45: 363–95.

Cahill, M. (1994) *The New Social Policy*, Oxford: Basil Blackwell.

Cole, G. (1999) 'All-in-one but not one-for-all', *Financial Times*, 23 February 1999.

Conaty, P. and Mayo, E. (1997) *A Commitment to People and Place: the Case for Community Development Credit Unions*, London: New Economics Foundation.

Credit Card Research Group (1998) *What's On the Cards?* London: Credit Card Research Group.

Cruickshank, D. (2000) *Competition in UK Banking: a Report to the Chancellor of the Exchequer*, London: HMSO.

Financial Services Authority (1998) *Promoting Public Understanding of Financial Services: a Strategy for Consumer Education*, London: Financial Services Authority.

Ford, J. (1991) *Consuming Credit: Debt and Poverty in the UK*, London: Child Poverty Action Group.

Goode, J., Callender, C. and Lister, R. (1998) *Purse or Wallet? Gender Inequalities and Income Distribution within Families on Benefits*, London: Policy Studies Institute.

Ibison, D., Newman, C. and Tighe, C. (2000) 'Barclays in political tangle over closure plan', *Financial Times*, 5 April, p. 3.

Ibison, D. (2000) 'High street "villain" takes the flak for the big four', *Financial Times*, 5 April, p. 3.

Kempson, E. (1994) *Outside the Banking System: a Review of Households without a Current Account*, London: HMSO.

Kempson, E. and Whyley, C. (1999) *Kept out or Opted out: Understanding and Combating Financial Exclusion*, Bristol: Policy Press.

Knight, D. and Odih, P. (1995) 'It's about time: the significance of gendered time for financial services consumption', *Time and Society*, 4(2): 205–31.

Laurie, H. (1996) *Women's Employment Decisions and Financial Arrangements within the Household*, Ph.D. Thesis: University of Essex.

Leyshon, A., Thrift, N. and Justice, M. (1993) *A Reversal of Fortune: Financial Services and the South East of England*, London: Seeds.

Lewis, A., Betts, H. and Webley, P. (1997) *Financial Services: a Literature Review of Consumer Attitudes, Preferences and Perceptions*, Bath: University of Bath School of Social Sciences.

Molloy, D. and Snape, D. (1999) *Low Income Households: Financial Organisation and Financial Exclusion – a Review of the Literature*, London: Department of Social Security.

Morris, L and Ruane, S. (1989) *Household Finance Management and the Labour Market*, Aldershot: Avebury.

National Consumer Council (1999) *Financial Services and Markets Bill Response to the Treasury's Consultation on the Draft Bill*, London: National Consumer Council.

Nyman, C. (1999) 'Gender equality in "the most equal country in the world": money and marriage in Sweden', *Sociological Review* 47(4): 766–93.

Office of National Statistics (1996) *Family Expenditure Survey*, London: HMSO.

Oppenheim, C. (1998) *An Inclusive Society: Strategies for Tackling Poverty*, London: Institute for Public Policy Research.

Pahl, J. (1989) *Money and Marriage*, London: Macmillan.

—— (1995) 'His money, her money: recent research on financial organisation in marriage', *Journal of Economic Psychology* 16(3): 361–76.

—— (1999) *Invisible Money: Family Finances in the Electronic Economy*, Bristol: The Policy Press.

Rowlingson, K. (1994) *Moneylenders and their Customers*, London: Policy Studies Institute.

Rowlingson, K. and Kempson, E. (1994) *Paying with Plastic: a Study of Credit Card Debt*, London: Policy Studies Institute.

Singh, S. (1997) *Marriage Money: the Social Shaping of Money in Marriage and Banking*, St Leonards, NSW, Australia: Allen and Unwin.

Singh, S and Ryan, A. (1999) *Gender, Design and Electronic Commerce*, Centre for International Research on Communication and Information Technologies, Melbourne: RMIT University.

Treasury Committee (1999a) *Third Report: Financial Services Regulation*, HC 1998–99 73–I, London: HMSO.

—— (1999b) *Third Report: Financial Services Regulation*, HC 1998–99 73–II, London: HMSO.

Vogler, C. (1998) 'Money in the household: some underlying issues of power', *Sociological Review* 46(4): 687–713.

Vogler, C. and Pahl, J. (1993) 'Social and economic change and the organisation of money in marriage', *Work, Employment and Society* 7(1): 71–95.

—— (1994) 'Money, power and inequality within marriage', *Sociological Review* 42(2): 263–88.

Wilson, G. (1987) *Money in the Family*, Aldershot: Avebury.

Chapter 6

Complex equalities
Redistribution, class and gender

Peter Taylor-Gooby

Background

Most people on the Left think more equality would be a good thing. Equality, however, is a can of worms, once people become aware that people can be unequal on more than one dimension. What for example would be the impact of greater gender equality on social class inequalities? What are the impacts on privilege and vulnerability in a society which has developed a (creaking) legal framework against gender discrimination, but does not have a mechanism to advance class equality, and which is a member of the EU, with its directives on Equal Treatment which cover gender but not class (or race)? This chapter analyses theoretical debates about gender, class and inequality and about the future of the welfare state. It uses material from the British Household Panel Survey (BHPS) to illustrate a discussion of what the consistent pursuit of egalitarianism might mean in modern social policy.

The theoretical debates about welfare have been influenced by arguments from a number of directions, including the economics of rational choice, the sociology of risk society and analyses of globalization, which have led to a revision of some long-standing assumptions about one-dimensional class equality in social policy, both as a feasible goal for government policy and as something that citizens see as particularly desirable in any case. One result is that inequalities along the lines of social class occupy less attention, as analysts become more aware of the importance of other dimensions of inequality. Another is that, for a variety of reasons, the capacity of government to promote equality is seen as more limited.

Approaches to inequality: new directions in welfare theory

The traditional Left were concerned with inequality along the dimension of class, and with outcomes rather than processes, so that the goal was the reduction of inequalities between social classes. In recent years, our understanding of policy has become responsive to the complexity of inequality along independent but intersecting dimensions, (see for example, the path-breaking work of Fiona Williams (1992) and Ruth Lister's discussion of 'differentiated universalism'

(1997, ch. 3)). In addition, the main left party in the UK has shifted its stance from a concern with equality of outcome towards equality of opportunity – for example, one influential figure writes: 'The Left . . . has in the past too readily downplayed its duty to provide a wide range of opportunities for individuals to advance themselves . . . At worst, it has stifled opportunity in the name of abstract equality' (Blair 1998: 3). The interaction between equality of outcome and of opportunity has been extensively discussed (see for example, Crosland (1956), Barry (1990), Plant (1984)). This chapter analyses recent theoretical discussion of welfare policy to understand how the shift has come about. It then goes on to investigate whether there is a conflict between policies designed to promote equality of outcome and those concerned with gender inequalities and, if so, how the conflict should be resolved.

The issue is highlighted by two facts and is relevant to recent developments in social policy debate. The two facts are as follows: first, income inequality in the UK has grown sharply in recent years (Goodman, Johnson and Webb 1997: 112) at a time when, on some measures, gender inequalities of income are growing somewhat smaller. Thus average women's wage rates – the rates for each hour of work – have risen to just over 80 per cent of men's from 69 per cent in 1985, but earnings lag behind at 72 per cent, up from 62 per cent, because women tend to spend, on average, fewer hours than men in formal employment (CSO 1999: 92, Lonsdale 1987: 96). Second, there is a tendency for men and women to partner with others in related social and income positions, so that there is a strong correlation between partners' individual and household income. The Pearson correlation between personal income and household income for those in full-time work in the 1997 BHPS is 0.67 for women and 0.81 for men (significant at the 1 per cent level). Even across the 300-odd categories of the standard occupational classification represented in the survey, the correlation is 0.34 (significant at the 1 per cent level).

Since class is related to life chances and to income and many of the (justified) demands for equal treatment in pay concern claims that women should receive rewards closer to the higher rewards typically commanded by men, it is plausible that movement towards greater income equality between women and men might lead to greater income *in*equality between households. This would result as women and men would tend to receive incomes that are more equal within social class groups and tend also to partner within those groups. Inequality would fall between women and men within those groups, but would increase between the groups. Thus progressive policies designed to promote gender equality might come into conflict with progressive policies designed to promote class equality. Conversely, if equality were advanced by lowering men's incomes to the level currently experienced by women, inequalities between households might be reduced – a strategy whose electoral implications Left government in an affluent society might wish to consider! Whichever way the argument runs, it is clear that gender and class inequality must be considered at the same time, if policies followed for the best of egalitarian motives are not to produce unintended consequences. There is a problem if New Labour simply abandons the traditional Left concern with class inequality.

The new approaches to welfare policy are more complex, but require considera-tion in some depth, because they provide the underpinning to the new directions in policy-making that take the emphasis away from issues of redistribution, whether on class or gender lines. Dominant strands in policy ideas now current tend to minimize the importance of class inequality, and thus divert attention from discussion of developments that might increase such inequality. Class differences in life chances are low on the New Labour agenda. The central claims are that the capacity of welfare states to promote greater equality through redistributive measures is weakened by factors beyond the control of governments. Even if government were in a position to pursue such aims, citizens are no longer as interested in the promotion of equality as they once were. We will examine rational choice theory as applied to welfare and also the influence of the more sociological theories of risk society on New Labour 'Third Way' thinking. What these approaches have in common is that they see both people's ideas about their interests and the scope of welfare policy as more individualistic, leading to the view that policy is and should be more a matter of individual opportunity and less a matter of outcomes.

Rational choice in welfare policy debate

In a path-breaking paper, Julian Le Grand (1997) identifies four groups of actors centrally involved in the operation of the welfare state – the politicians who propose and enact legislation and raise taxes and contributions, the state officials and professionals who manage and deliver services, the citizen/taxpayers who finance the services and the service users who rely on state provision (see Figure 6.1). The post-war welfare settlement assumed a combination of deference and passivity on the part of the citizens and altruism and activity on the part of politicians and planners. Those who made and managed welfare policy would act in the common interest and the taxpayers would be content to pay what was demanded, while service users would accept the provision and priority orders that were offered to them.

The new approach in welfare policy-making finds its intellectual basis in rational choice theory derived ultimately from the economics of consumption. This approach has been influenced by the work of Schumpeter (1944), Niskanen (1973) and Downs (1957) on political and bureaucratic behaviour; Breton (1974) and Buchanan and Tullock (1962) on taxpayers' behaviour and Murray (1984) and Mead (1986) on the behaviour of service users. The central claim of the rational choice perspective is that behaviour can be understood in terms of the selection between alternatives on the grounds of the balance of advantage over cost. This approach sees political activity as dominated by the support of voters for policies which benefit their own group and the response of politicians and parties in offering policy platforms designed to appeal on this basis to a winning constituency. It sees administrative activity as dominated by the desire of officials to maximize their own interests by expanding their empire (or, in more recent times, by being at the

	Traditional model	Rational choice model
Politicians and planners	altruistic/active (acts in public interest)	self-interested/proactive (seeks favour of voters)
Managers and professionals	altruistic/active (pursues service user interest)	self-interested/proactive (seeks to enlarge bureau/budget)
Citizens as taxpayers	Deferential/passive (happy to pay the set taxes)	self-interested/proactive (tax revolt)
Citizens as service users	deferential/passive (accepts standards and priorities)	self-interested/proactive (challenges provision, jumps queues, cheats on benefits)

Figure 6.1   From altruism+deference to self-interest+proactivity

Source: Based on Le Grand 1997

forefront in implementing and managing cuts), and the actions of ordinary citizens as being determined by enthusiasm for policies which will maximize their interests and minimize the taxes they pay. Correspondingly, the government can no longer assume that the pattern of services and priorities it lays down will be passively accepted by service users; individuals will increasingly act to maximize their own advantage. Individuals will (it is supposed) seek to use their social skills, cultural capital or capacity to move house to the best serviced areas to gain privileged access to professionals or the most attractive services, thus confounding attempts to set priorities. Benefit claimers may manage their social security entitlement, for example, fraudulently claiming unemployment benefit whilst working or disability benefits while able-bodied.

The model which links proactivity and self-interest as the basis of behaviour is often assumed to undermine the traditional welfare state. It is important because it appears to be extremely influential in guiding government thinking, particularly in the more liberal European regimes, notably New Labour, and hence in supporting welfare retrenchment. The question arises of why this transition in the intellectual approach which underlies policy-making has taken place. What social changes have provided the space for the incursion of the rational choice approach? New sociological theories provide accounts of the ideological shifts. These theories argue that the dominant trends in welfare citizenship are a growing mistrust of the government's capacity to meet citizen needs and an increasingly confident proactive stance by service users that undermines reliance on the state. They account for these developments in terms of risk society, globalization and social diversity.

Risk and good government

Beck's *Risk Society*, originally published at the time of Chernobyl, was pivotal in drawing attention to the importance of 'manufactured risk'. The claim is that, while risk and uncertainty remain continuing features of human life (a point which Beck may not sufficiently emphasize, though it is certainly made by Giddens – for example (1994: 21), recent developments have imported a new perspective into the perception and understanding of risk. In traditional society, risk was due primarily to the operation of natural forces or of external human interventions perceived as analogous to natural forces (plague, drought, the barbarians at the gate). The modern perception of risk includes the awareness that human interventions into nature (through technological innovation – for example genetic modification) and into society (through government policies or economic activities – town planning, industrial subsidy) may also generate damage. The argument is clearest in the fields of interventions in the environment (acid rain, global warming, the Oklahoma dust-bowl), biochemistry or pharmacology (Thalidomide). However many aspects of modern industrial systems generate welfare needs and problems including unemployment, housing needs and the cessation of income from employment as a result of technological change.

The point here is not that the complex empirical balance of benefit and damage from human activity is negative, but rather that it is irredeemably uncertain – and that people are increasingly aware of this. A more highly educated and better informed citizenry understands that many activities have generated unintended risks in the past. The future impact of current interventions is unknown and is modelled in radically different ways. The abolition of school selection, waste disposal, transport, food irradiation, pension policy, membership of EMU, support for one-parent families and introduction of the minimum wage are currently the stuff of political debate because there is no expert consensus about what the impact of proposed changes might be. The qualitatively distinctive feature of modern times is that we no longer trust expert opinion or the results of impartial scientific inquiry because scientifically based plans and the deployment of technology have let us down so many times in the past. Risk is endemic in the modern world. The decisions of government and of experts are continuously open to question by an increasingly more knowledgeable and informed public.

The interchange of ideas and the shifts in economic focus due to globalization provide further challenges to state authority.

Globalization

Globalization includes both economic and cultural aspects. The claim that government can exert an effective economic control of the national economy has been seriously damaged by the growing importance of centres of economic power outside the traditional welfare states and by the rapid expansion of international competition, so that the proportion of GNP that is traded internationally is returning to the levels of the imperialist era (Hirst and Thompson 1996).

The expansion of international trade, the dissolution of the political barriers imposed by the communist/capitalist split and the growing role of new capitalist countries also influence policy. Much of the debate has concerned newly-industrialized Asian economies. Available evidence indicates that Asian exports make up a relatively small proportion of European imports, but have succeeded in capturing from Europe much of the growth in developing markets elsewhere in Asia and in Africa (Held *et al.* 1999, Table 3.6). The proportion of European and US trade made up of low-cost Southern imports is estimated to have doubled between the late 1970s and the early 1990s (Wood 1994; Esping-Andersen 1995: 256–61). The former state socialist nations of Central and Eastern Europe are strong competitors for West European investment and trade.

The second factor diminishing national economic control is the growth in multinational companies and political institutions alongside the freer international markets. Multinational corporations have expanded very rapidly over the past fifteen years (Mishra 1999: 49). One recent estimate is that about two-fifths of the jobs created by British-origin multinationals are abroad (Marginson 1994: 64). Nations which wish to attract or retain investment from such companies experience competitive pressures in relation to state policies in the areas mentioned above and these must affect their capacity to pursue independent welfare policies (Mishra 1999, ch. 2). The importance of political institutions such as the EU with its Single European Market and the recently established North American Free Trade Association is at present hard to judge. Some writers argue that the EU's role in economic policy-making already constitutes it as a kind of multi-tiered federal state (Leibfried and Pierson 1995) while others believe that 'it is difficult to see how a close union can be achieved unless new or complementary institutions for delivery of social protection are devised' (Begg and Nectoux 1995: 300).

Cultural globalization extends the economic notion of globalization to refer to the impact of improvements in communication whereby individuals in any part of the world can be aware of developments elsewhere on the planet, almost simultaneously, just as their material interests are directly influenced by economic developments elsewhere. This change has profound implications for the way we live our lives. Giddens refers to the process whereby traditional frameworks of time and space are dissolved, and argues that cultural globalization contributes to the erosion of traditional social structures:

> Globalization should not just be seen as an 'out there' phenomenon, but as an 'in here' one also: it affects not only localities but even intimacies of personal existence since it acts to transform everyday life . . . thus for instance the emergence of local nationalisms, and an accentuating of local identities, are bound up with globalizing influences to which they stand in opposition.
>
> (Giddens 1994: 23)

In this context the unified structure of interests that supported the traditional models of state welfare is subject to fragmentation.

Social diversity

People's interests become more diverse. In relation to the sphere of work, there is greater insecurity in working life as a result of more complex patterns of competition (associated with globalization and with technical developments) and more far-reaching industrial planning, and the entry of new groups of workers in larger numbers; family structures are more diverse due to greater control over fertility, longer life expectancy, more divorce and more expression of sexual preferences. At the same time a wider range of spheres of social activity have become politicized so that political struggles no longer simply concern distributional issues mainly along the lines of social class, but increasingly are involved with issues of ecology, sexual, ethnic or regional identity, community interests, disability or age.

These three developments – risk society, globalization and greater social diversity – all in their different ways call into question the traditional patterns of governmental authority and imply that the assumptions that fostered the structure of a top-down bureaucratic welfare state can no longer be sustained.

Reflexivity and political consciousness

In work that has arguably influenced policy-thinking among New Labour (Giddens 2000), Giddens links the mistrust of expertise and of traditional authority to globalization and diversity to claim that a transformation in political consciousness is taking place. He combines these arguments with theories which foreground changes in social consciousness as the motor of transition. He identifies three developments as important in determining responses to the awareness of risk, the growth of economic insecurity and the weakness of traditional welfare state solutions to it: (i) globalization, both in terms of economic interconnection and also the 'complex mix of interacting local, national and global processes affecting trade, lifestyle, consciousness and identity' (Giddens 1994: 4), (ii) the emergence of a post-traditional order in which traditional patterns of behaviour and institutions are continually open to interrogation and the requirement that they must justify themselves, and (iii) the increasing importance of social reflexivity.

Since people are better informed than ever, less inclined to put a blind trust in government, experts or in tradition, and live increasingly diverse lifestyles which result in priority being directed to different issues, they must take greater responsibility for developing their own solutions to the problems they experience. If existentialists argued that we are 'condemned to be free', this perspective may suggest that we are condemned to the new individualism (see Figure 6.2).

Individuals are increasingly aware of the range both of expert opinion and of cultural practice on issues ranging from individual lifestyle and relationships to the operation of the political economy, and of the fact that they can rely on no one to sift it for them. This reflexivity of social consciousness can be understood as a world of 'clever people' who are proactive: 'information produced by specialists

Risk	'Manufactured uncertainty' as 'a result of human intervention' into society or nature, not natural forces
Globalization	'Action at a distance' affects 'identity, consciousness, trade, lifestyle'
Post-traditional order	'Tradition is open to interrogation' – opposed to fundamentalism
Social reflexivity	'Clever' people who have access to information previously under 'expert' control, and mistrust experts, officials and traditional authority.

Figure 6.2 From modernism to post-modernism

Source: Based on Giddens 1994: 3–6

. . . can no longer be wholly confined to specific groups, but becomes routinely interpreted and acted upon by lay individuals in the course of their everyday actions' (Giddens 1994: 24).

The new perspective implies a change in the perceptions of the role of government in promoting welfare. In the past the legitimacy of the welfare state was bound up with its capacity to satisfy recognized needs. Now, while needs multiply for some groups and society is richer than ever, confidence in the capacity of the welfare state to meet them through its traditional strategies is in decline.

Implications for the welfare state

Arguments from two directions – the economics of rational choice and the sociology of risk society – combine to produce a common account of the contemporary welfare policy context that may be summed up in two points:

- Government capacity to undertake 'social engineering' to promote equality is now limited.
- More pro-active and individualized citizens would not necessarily wish it to do so in any case.

The traditional welfare state is dead. Under these circumstances the ideology of the Third Way in Welfare, which stresses a retreat by government, strict limits to intervention and substitution of equality of opportunity for equality of outcome (Blair 1998; Giddens 1998, 2000) advances. Old Labour debates about redistribution and equalizing life chances for different social classes disappear from the agenda. Greater equality of opportunity in the labour market is promoted, and legal rather than interventionist actions in this direction are pursued. If this is so, the question of whether limited advances in gender equality are associated with greater class inequality drops out of the ambit of policy debate. However the relation between inequalities in these spheres is of importance for two reasons. First, if action to advance the one damages the other, a contradiction in policy goals

– and in the constituencies for action – emerges. Second, society is growing increasingly unequal along the dimensions of individual and household income. Policies to advance gender equality must operate in the context of that trend and seek ways to mitigate it.

The impact of such policies in the future is to some extent a matter of speculation. However, evidence on current patterns of inequality is relevant. Moreover, such evidence can be analysed in order to extrapolate how equality might develop under controlled assumptions about the effect of current directions in policy. We move on to consider the evidence and its implications for policy development. Does the entirely justified (and sluggish) move towards greater gender equality, imply more class inequality?

Class, gender and income

Table 6.1 opposite gives information on income patterns across social classes, referring only to women and men in full-time work, to avoid the problems in comparison that may arise because women are more likely to work part-time. Thus the differences between men's and women's patterns of income in different social groups in the table cannot be attributed to differences in engagement in the formal labour market. The study uses the 1997 British Household Panel Survey, which provides a convenient high-quality data set. BHPS is a longitudinal survey, which seeks to re-interview the same individuals each year and trace the development of their lives. We are here using the 1997 data as an annual snapshot survey. The initial BHPS sample was nearly 10,000, but, due to the attrition normal in a survey of this kind, only about 7,000 cases were available as a fully-representative national sample for that year. In our analysis we use only women and men in full-time work which reduces the number of cases further, but still leaves adequate numbers for analysis. The survey is the best currently available source for charting the impact of the risks of modern life on people's living standards in the UK.

The table shows that, among the population in full-time work, women are over-represented among lower grade service class, routine non-manual and personal service workers and under-represented in all other groups, most strikingly among skilled manual and the higher grade service class. In every category listed, with the exception of personal service workers, women tend to earn less than men. This pattern has been extensively discussed elsewhere (for example, Crompton 1993: 93–7). It is hardly surprising that it makes a considerable contribution to the differences in the income distribution of women and men. Table 6.2 shows the patterns of income inequality among women and men full-time workers. They are clearly similar, but with a markedly lower mean among women. The distribution is also more positively skewed among women – with a rather greater concentration at the bottom end, a difference mainly accounted for by the greater access of men to high paid jobs. Note again that the table refers to those in full-time work (30 hours plus) only, so that the picture here is not directly affected by the greater participation of women in part-time work.

Table 6.1 Income by Hope-Goldthorpe class and sex, those in full-time work

	Women		Men		Women's income as % of men's
	Mean income (£)	%	Mean income (£)	%	%
Service class, higher grade	23399	14.6	29147	20.4	80.3
Service class, lower grade	15882	29.0	20685	19.1	76.8
Routine non-manual	11383	26.5	14971	5.8	76.0
Personal service workers	9025	7.3	8521	0.9	105.9
Small proprietors with employees	15266	1.7	20458	3.7	74.6
Small proprietors without employees	10863	1.9	14204	8.1	76.5
Foremen, Technicians	10024	4.0	16732	9.8	60.6
Skilled manual	9122	2.7	14202	12.6	64.2
Semi/Unskilled manual	8566	11.9	12317	18.0	69.5
N	1498		2539		4037

Source: British Household Panel Survey , 1997

Table 6.2 Average income per decile for women, men and households

	Women (£)	Men (£)	Households (£)
Ist decile	4696	6165	5163
2nd	7425	10507	8463
3rd	9000	12576	10474
4th	10440	14310	12101
5th	11709	16123	13762
6th	13115	17960	15660
7th	15006	20580	17831
8th	17562	23253	20866
9th	21424	27517	24746
10th	32036	43640	38675

Source: British Household Panel Survey, 1997

The factors which explain this pattern are many. They include discrimination against women in promotion and in access to better-paid work, 'glass-ceiling' effects, the inadequate operation of EU Equal Treatment directives and national equal pay and sex discrimination legislation in the UK, traditions which link the female gender to work in lower-paid sectors and which depress pay in those sectors, interrupted career patterns, male demands for women to devote time to families and unwillingness to take an equal share in the domestic work whose product they enjoy and the differential impact of care responsibilities for children and dependent adults on women. Nonetheless, movement towards greater equality between the sexes in the labour market is an objective endorsed in the governing party's election manifesto (Labour Party 1997: 25) and some limited progress in this direction has been made, as the evidence on wage and earnings differentials given earlier shows. How far this progress results from policy and how far it is the outcome of changes in the labour market and in family patterns beyond the control of government is unclear.

The impact of greater gender equality on household inequality

The survey data may be used to investigate the primary practical question with which this chapter is concerned: the likely impact of greater gender equality on household income inequalities in this country. Surveys such as BHPS are most frequently analysed to provide information on existing social patterns among those interviewed – to reflect, as it were, a representative image of society. However they may also be used to examine the hypothetical situation that might exist were society to differ in some respect – as a crystal ball, rather than a mirror. This can be done by altering the variable that measures the characteristic we are interested in within the data set to create, as it were, the survey that would have been produced had society differed in the way we define, but in no other way. The data set generated by this manipulation is the data that would be produced by a survey under such hypothetical circumstances. It thus provides a convenient way of studying social changes, analogous to a thought experiment.

In this case, the method used is to construct hypothetical measures of income distribution which reflect what the pattern of income inequality in society would be like, were women to be paid the same as men and vice versa. These may then be compared with the existing income distribution. Variables are computed in which women's average income in each Hope Goldthorpe class group is substituted for that of each class group for men and vice versa.[1] These variables retain the number of cases of one sex which exist in the survey sample (thus representing proportionately the class structure of the country by sex) but attribute to that sex the income of the members of the other sex in the corresponding class group. The variables are then substituted for the existing women's and existing men's contribution to total household income as appropriate. In the case of the women interviewed, men's average income in each category is used for each social class category of women and the converse procedure carried for the men interviewed.

This procedure generates hypothetical distributions, which represent circumstances in which women are paid the same as men and are now in each of the Hope-Goldthorpe social classes, and vice versa. These imaginary worlds – women paid like men and men paid like women – may be compared with the existing distributions for the households of which each woman and each man interviewed is a member, and with each other. It is of course unlikely that income distribution will evolve so that men's pay distribution becomes the same as that currently endured by women, or vice versa. However the 'thought experiment' may describe two limiting conditions – 'men as women' and 'women as men', between which the future development of incomes may plausibly lie. The models are valuable because they give an insight into what a more gender-equal world might be like in terms of household income distribution.

Table 6.3 shows the results of the computation. The analysis is again confined to households containing married or cohabiting couples in which both partners are in full-time work, in order to ensure that the impact of part-time work on incomes does not distort the class effect. It gives the mean income of the various household groups and information about the patterns of the distribution. Thus the impact of shifting women's incomes to men (and vice versa) on both the absolute level of household income and on the relative degree of inequality between top and bottom can be judged.

Unsurprisingly, the hypothetical households in which the component provided by women's incomes is set to that of men in corresponding class groups have a higher mean than the current distribution, because both partners now have access to men's higher incomes, while those in which men's contribution is set to that of women by social class is lower. The skew is greater in column 1 than in column 3, but not so high as columns 2 and 4 in which the small number of high earning men affects the measure. The share of the top 20 and bottom 40 per cent also

Table 6.3 Household income distribution for the women interviewed on the assumption that women's incomes become the same as men's are now and vice versa, and the current distribution for the households of which they form part, full-time employed only

	Households: women's incomes at level of men	Current distribution, households of women interviewed	Households: men's incomes at level of women	Current distribution, households of men interviewed
Mean	£39613	£35687	£30845	£35813
Standard deviation	£15096	£17414	£12646	£17602
Skew	2.33	2.54	1.87	2.59
% share of top 20%	31.0	30.9	32.2	30.2
% share of bottom 40%	27.9	28.2	26.4	30.1
Coefficient of variation	0.07	0.12	0.08	0.12
N	723	725	738	742

Source: British Household Panel Survey, 1997

stretches slightly in the 'men as women', rather than in the 'women as men' households. However none of the differences are very large.

The distribution of women's and men's incomes does not differ greatly in shape but does differ in level. The mean household incomes of the samples we examine are currently about £35,000. If men's incomes are reduced to the level of women's in corresponding class groups, the household income falls to about £31,000. If women's incomes rise to the level of men's, average household income rises to about £40,000. However, the overall shape of the distribution remains broadly similar in both cases. Paying women the same as men, and vice versa, would not make a very substantial difference to the *degree* of inequality, but would certainly affect the *level* of household incomes.

Conclusion

These findings have important implications for progressive policies in a context where government is more passive and citizens more active. This is the context of modern policy-making, as the theoretical debates reviewed earlier and their influence on New Labour imply. Equality in principle could be advanced by moving women's incomes closer to men's (in most cases effectively levelling up) or moving men's closer to women's (levelling down). The likely impact of equal opportunity legislation leads in both directions – women gain increases by using men as comparators, while changes in the labour market, including the greater participation of women, create competitive pressures that move men closer to women. The hypothetical experiment indicates that the main impact of the shift to gender equality on household income is on the level of income rather than on class inequalities. There is no strong conflict between the promotion of greater gender equality by levelling up and class inequalities.

The good news is that the view that social inequality (at a household level) on class lines would grow markedly wider, were gender equality in pay to be achieved and women's pay to rise to the level of men's, is incorrect (compare columns 1 and 2 in Table 6.3). The relative pattern of inequality would stay more or less the same. The bad news (at least for the traditional Left) is that it is also true that such a policy would do nothing for the current pattern of class inequalities. Households would remain roughly as unequal in a relative sense, but inequalities would of course grow larger in an absolute sense, while remaining relatively the same, because the class inequalities in men's pay are absolutely larger than those in women's and these inequalities would now operate more broadly across both genders. How does this relate to the theoretical and policy debates with which we started?

The implications of the evidence may be stated simply. The arguments that the state is no longer in a position, whether as a result of shifts in the context in which it operates due to globalization, or shifts in public support due to rational choices and reflexivity, to pursue interventionism in favour of greater equality of outcomes require re-examination. If Left governments believe that it is no longer a practical proposition to advance equality of outcomes, and limit themselves to the pursuit of equality of opportunity, so that opportunities for women to gain incomes gradually improve, then the current slow move to gender equality may continue, but in a way that simply sustains current patterns of household inequality. Equal opportunities and equal incomes for women and men will certainly tackle the injustices associated with the long-standing tradition of discrimination against women, but will neither increase nor reduce the inequalities between households. The point is that a government which wishes to tackle inequalities between households must pursue policies which deal with some of the traditional concerns of the Left, the class inequalities in income which affect both men and women. This takes us beyond an approach which disregards the significance of social class. The recognition that inequality is not one-dimensional is an important advance in the social analysis that underpins welfare debate. New approaches designed to tackle a broader range of inequalities through policies concerned primarily with opportunity rather than outcome must not lose sight of the continuing significance of the old class inequalities which were the staple of the traditional Left.

Notes

1   Averages of the income for women and for men in each of the nine Hope-Goldthorpe social class groups given in Table 6.1 (service class, higher grade; service class, lower grade; routine non-manual; and so on – see Goldthorpe and Hope 1974) were calculated.

Then the average for the men was substituted for the average for the women in each class group, so that service class higher grade women were treated as if they received the average salary of service class higher grade men and so on. This is a situation of hypothetical gender equality through levelling up. In a separate exercise the average incomes for each Hope-Goldthorpe class group for women were substituted for those of men, to give the hypothetical income distribution under conditions of gender equality, but with men's income levelled down to those of women. These computations enable us to examine what greater gender equality might imply on the assumption that women's incomes are levelled up and also on the assumption that men's incomes are levelled down.

References

Barry, N. (1990) *Welfare*, Milton Keynes: Open University Press.

Blair, T. (1998) *The Third Way*, pamphlet no 588, London: Fabian Society.

Beck, U., Giddens, A. and Lash, S. (1994) *Reflexive Modernisation*, Cambridge: Polity Press.

Begg, I. and Nectoux, F. (1995) 'Social Protection and European Union', *Journal of European Social Policy* 5(4): 285–302.

Breton, A. (1974) *The Economic Theory of Representative Government*, Basingstoke: Macmillan.

Buchanan, J. and Tullock, G. (1962) *The Calculus of Consent*, Ann Arbor: University of Michigan Press.

Commission of the EU (1994) *White Paper on European Social Policy*, Com (94) 333.

Commission on Social Justice (1994) *Social Justice: Strategies for national renewal*, London: Vintage.

Crompton, R. (1997) *Class and Stratification*, Oxford: Polity Press.

Crosland, A. (1956) *The Future of Socialism*, London: Jonathan Cape.

CSO (Central Statistical Office) (1999), *Social Trends no 29*, London: HMSO.

Downs, A. (1957) *An Economic Theory of Politics*, New York: Harper and Row.

Esping-Andersen, G. (1995) *Welfare States in Transition*, London: Sage.

Giddens, A. (1994) *Beyond Left and Right?* Cambridge: Polity Press.

—— (1998) *The Third Way*, Cambridge: Polity Press.

—— (2000) *The Third Way and Its Critics*, Cambridge: Polity Press.

Goldthorpe, J. and Hope, K. (1974) *The Social Grading of Occupations, a New Approach and Scale*, Oxford: Clarendon Press.

Goodman, A., Johnson, P. and Webb, S. (1997) *Inequality in the UK*, Oxford: Oxford University Press.

Held, D., McGrew, A., Goldblatt, D. and Perraton, J. (1999) *Global Transformations*, Cambridge: Polity Press.

Hirst, P. and Thompson, G. (1996) *Globalization in Question : the international and the possibilities of governance*, Cambridge: Polity Press.

Labour Party (1997) *New Labour: Because Britain Deserves Better*, Election Manifesto.

Le Grand, J. (1997) 'Knights, Knaves or Pawns? Human Behaviour and Social Policy', *Journal of Social Policy*, 26(2): 149–70.

Leibfried, S. and Pierson, P. (eds) (1995) *European Social Policy: between Fragmentation and Integration*, Washington: Brookings Institution.

Lister, R. (1997) *Citizenship: Feminist Perspectives*, Basingstoke: Macmillan.

Lonsdale, S. (1987) 'Patterns of Paid Work' in C. Glendinning and J. Millar (eds) *Women and Poverty in Britain*, Brighton: Harvester Wheatsheaf.

Marginson, P. (1994) 'Multinational Britain: employment and work in an internationalised economy', *Human Resource Management Journal*, 4(4): 63–80.

Mead, L. (1986) *Beyond Entitlement: the social obligations of citizenship*, New York: Free Press.

Mishra, R. (1999) *Globalisation and the Welfare State*, Cheltenham: Edward Elgar.

Murray, G. (1984) *Losing Ground: American social policy 1950–1980*, New York: Basic Books.

Niskanen, W. (1973) *Bureaucracy – Servant or Master?*, London: Institute of Economic Affairs.

Plant, R. (1984) *Equality, Markets and the State*, Fabian Tract 494, London: Fabian Society.

Schumpeter, J. (1976 [1944]) *Capitalism, Socialism and Democracy*, London: Allen and Unwin.

Williams, F. (1992) 'Somewhere over the rainbow: universality and diversity in social policy', in N. Manning and R. Page (1992) *Social Policy Review, 4*, Social Policy Association.

Wood, A. (1994) North–South Trade, *Employment and Inequality*, Oxford: Oxford University Press.

Chapter 7

'Work for those who can, security for those who cannot'

A third way in social security reform or fractured social citizenship?[1]

Ruth Lister

Introduction

Social security (aka welfare) reform is, as Tony Blair has made clear, central to the New Labour 'project'. The chapter begins with a brief discussion of the paradigm shift in Labour's thinking: from an equality agenda to one comprising the trinity of Responsibility, Inclusion and Opportunity (RIO), expressed primarily through paid work. This agenda stands at the heart of the 'new contract for welfare', representing a 'third way' in welfare reform, 'promoting opportunity instead of dependence' (DSS 1998: 19).

Overshadowed by the guiding principle of 'work for those who can, security for those who cannot', more traditional debates about benefit adequacy and the overall structure of social security, and in particular the balance between meanstested and non-meanstested benefits, are dismissed as irrelevant and old-fashioned. The chapter will argue, though, that they cannot be ignored, if 'security for those who cannot' is to be treated as seriously as 'work for those who can' in the implementation of social security reform. In the absence of public debate about the reform of the structure of social security, the danger is that individual policy changes will add up to a significant shift in the 'welfare regime' mix further towards the liberal model. The implications for the fabric of citizenship and for the security of a significant proportion of the population are potentially profound.

The failure to give equal priority to the 'security' side of the work–security equation reflects, in part, a false dichotomy upon which much New Labour discussion of welfare reform is based. In contrast, as the chapter will go on to argue, the more general notion of a 'third way' sets up the false alternatives of 'Old Left' and 'New Right' (as the only existing alternatives). This provides the basis for a false synthesis, in that it glosses over a genuine political dichotomy, which reflects the continued power of social divisions. Finally, in conclusion, the chapter will explore briefly a dissonance which is beginning to emerge between aspects of the rhetoric of the third way and the reality of practical policies.

The new agenda of RIO

The legacy of eighteen years of New Right Conservative Government was, above all, an ideological one. As Driver and Martell put it: 'what New Labour has become is defined by Thatcherism'. Its response is 'an exercise in post-Thatcherite politics' (1998: 3, 1), shaped by Thatcherism yet also representing a reaction against it. It is a politics couched in the language of social justice, but a less egalitarian conceptualization of social justice than hitherto and one which, arguably, is overshadowed by a concern (albeit less explicit) with social cohesion that underpins RIO.

During the Conservative years, social security reform was driven by the objectives of promoting independence and individual and family responsibility; 'targeting' help on those in greatest need; improving work incentives and combating fraud and 'abuse'. Their overall effect was to increase the proportion of social security spending devoted to means-testing and to increase private welfare responsibility in its different dimensions of the market, voluntary sector and family. The complex mix that comprises the British 'welfare regime' was shifted decisively in the direction of the liberal model. The material legacy of these changes, combined with regressive taxation and labour market policies in the context of an increasingly fissured labour market, was a country scarred by a level of inequality exceptional by both post-war and international standards.

The themes running through Conservative social security policy live on in New Labour's welfare reform lexicon. In contrast to the Conservatives, however, New Labour does identify the overall increase in income inequality as a problem. Nevertheless, and despite continued vestiges of Labour's traditional vision of a more equal society, there has been a marked retreat from greater equality as an explicit goal and from redistribution through the tax–benefit system as the primary mechanism for achieving it. In their place, the emphasis now is on 'redistribution of opportunity' through education, training and paid employment.

This shift in focus from greater 'equality of outcomes' to 'equality of opportunity' and from redistribution of resources to what Tony Giddens calls 'redistribution of possibilities' (1998: 101) is widely seen as definitive of Third Way thinking. Likewise Giddens explains, the new Third Way politics 'defines equality as inclusion and inequality as exclusion' (1998: 102). Some commentators question, though, whether genuine inclusion in such an unequal society is possible without greater redistribution than the Government is prepared to contemplate.

New Labour's analysis of and prescription for tackling social exclusion is rooted in a belief that paid work is the primary route to social inclusion, reflecting what Ruth Levitas (1998) calls a 'social integrationist discourse'. This discourse is also reflected in the emphasis on responsibility that is central to the construction of the Third Way. Indeed Giddens, in his exposition of the Third Way, goes so far as to propose '*no rights without responsibilities*' as '*a prime motto for the new politics*' (Giddens, 1998: 65, emphasis in original).

Through a discourse of responsibilities and obligations, Blair has set out to reorient the Party's understanding of citizenship. In his own Third Way statement for the Fabian Society, he argues that 'for too long, the demand for rights from the state was separated from the duties of citizenship and the imperative for mutual responsibility on the part of individuals and institutions' (Blair 1998a: 4). Back in 1995, he distanced himself from 'early Left thinking' in which the 'language of responsibility [was] spoken far less fluently' than that of rights. He argued for a two-way covenant of duties between society and citizens which 'allows us to be much tougher and hard-headed in the rules we apply; and how we apply them' (1995). This 'hard-headedness' can be found in a range of social policy areas, most notably social security, but also anti-social behaviour and crime and disorder, where the emphasis is on the responsibilities of families and parents.[2]

Blair's emphasis on responsibilities reflects an ideological eclecticism which draws on a number of influences, including popular communitarianism, Christian Socialism and social liberalism (Deacon 1997; Beer 1998; Freeden 1999). Critics point to the dangers of an imbalance in the allocation of responsibilities and rights in an unequal society. Will Hutton, for example, while accepting a link between rights and obligations, has commented that 'most of the obligations that accompany rights in a New Labour order are shouldered by the bottom of society rather than those at the top, which is let off largely scot-free' (*The Observer*, 5 July 1998; see also, Fitzpatrick 1998). Thus, for example, there is no talk of taxation of the better off as an expression of citizenship responsibility to balance the emphasis on work obligations for those at the bottom.

'Reforming welfare around the work ethic'

Work, or to be more precise paid work, lies at the heart of the New Labour trinity of Responsibility, Inclusion and Opportunity, as reflected in the mantra 'reforming welfare around the work ethic'. The evils of 'welfare dependency' are a common refrain in the RIO discourses of New Labour, as they were under the Tories, despite the lack of empirical evidence to support the notion of a 'dependency culture' (Lister 1996; Bennett and Walker 1998). In both cases, the fingerprints of US New Right thinkers can be discerned.

As an antidote to 'welfare dependency', the obligation on benefit claimants to take up opportunities for paid work and training is stressed continually by ministers. The vehicle for exercising these obligations is the Government's flagship New Deal 'welfare to work' policy, to be implemented by a new 'welfare to work' agency, combining the former Benefit Agency and Employment Service. The New Deal is underpinned by social security reform, which combines 'sticks' and 'carrots'. On the 'carrot' side, there is the series of measures designed 'to make work pay' including the working families tax credit,[3] reform of national insurance contributions and the introduction of a minimum wage (albeit at a level lower than campaigned for by trade unions and the 'poverty lobby').

Under the Conservatives, the 'stick' applied to unemployed benefit claimants had become progressively tougher. Labour has taken the process further, with punitive penalties for those who do not comply with the compulsory New Deal schemes, and also benefit sanctions against workless offenders who fail to comply with community sentences. In addition, virtually all claimants of working age will now be expected to attend interviews with a personal adviser to discuss the prospects of finding work, as a condition of receiving benefit.

The new obligation to attend interviews was announced in language that was both revealing and disturbing. There were to be 'no apologies' for 'our tough benefits regime'. The Social Security Secretary, Alistair Darling, repeatedly underlined that fifty years on from the birth of the post-war welfare state, 'no one has an unqualified right to benefit' (*The Independent*, 10 February 1999). In the *Daily Mail*, Tony Blair explained that the reforms epitomise 'the new ethic of rights and responsibilities at the heart of our welfare state', summed up as the 'end of a something-for-nothing welfare state' (10 February 1999).

The New Deal reflects a broad consensus that paid employment does represent the best route out of poverty for those able to take it, and, as such, is to be welcomed. However, some commentators question the effectiveness of a strategy which focuses on employability rather than employment, as demand-side policies to reduce unemployment have effectively been abandoned in the face of the constraints believed to be imposed by globalizing economic forces. This reliance on 'supply-side' strategies alone is a particular concern in those parts of the country where there are not enough jobs for the various groups covered by the New Deal, who tend to be concentrated in the same low-employment areas (Turok and Webster 1998, Turok and Edge 1999). This criticism is only partially addressed by the New Deal for Communities, which is pursuing intensive regeneration in a number of the most deprived areas.

A more fundamental criticism is of the underlying philosophical premises of 'welfare to work', relating to the nature of paid work. The first is that paid work within a profoundly unequal labour market can necessarily be equated with social inclusion. The second is that it represents the primary obligation for all those of working age, discounting the value of community and voluntary activities and the unpaid work of reproduction and care carried out in the home, mainly still by women (Levitas 1998).

From the perspective of gender equity, the model pursued is primarily (though not unequivocally) that described by Nancy Fraser as 'the universal breadwinner model' of citizenship, in which the breadwinner role is universalized so that women can be citizen-workers alongside men (Fraser 1997; Fitzpatrick 1998). The launch of a child care strategy, as an integral part of economic policy, comprising both child care provision and family friendly employment policies, can be seen as supporting the universal breadwinner model. The refusal, hitherto, to introduce *paid* parental leave is indicative of a lack of commitment to an alternative 'universal caregiver' model, identified by Fraser, under which both men and women would be supported as citizen-earner/carers and carer/earners.[4] Nevertheless, for all the strategy's limitations, including those of resources, the symbolic importance of government recognition, in the UK, as in Continental Europe, that child care is, at least partially, a public responsibility is not to be underestimated.

Lone mothers taking up paid work are targeted as among the main beneficiaries of the child care strategy, in the face of evidence suggesting that lack of affordable and suitable child care acts as a major barrier to lone mothers' employment. It is in relation to lone mothers that the Government's work-biased approach has come under greatest criticism, despite broad support for policies that make it easier for them to move into paid work, if they want to. The decision to implement the Tory plan to abolish additional benefits for lone parents (originally proposed as a means of supporting the institution of marriage) was justified in part with reference to the paid work opportunities opened up by the New Deal and the child care strategy. This was interpreted by many lone mothers and their supporters as a denial of the importance of the unpaid work they do caring for their children which, research suggests, some lone mothers prioritize over paid work as more consistent with good mothering, at least while their children are young (Ford 1996; Duncan and Edwards 1999).

The Government can claim to support caring responsibilities through a range of policy initiatives. Yet, welcome as these are, they do not fully address what Levitas identifies as 'a profound contradiction between treating paid work as the defining factor in social inclusion, and recognising the value of unpaid work' (1998: 145). Underlying that contradiction is a narrow, gendered, interpretation of the obligations of citizenship (Lister 1997, 1999). Just as Western governments are placing increasing emphasis on paid work as the primary obligation of citizenship, a strong strand of feminist theorizing is advocating greater attention to care as an expression of citizenship responsibility. Selma Sevenhuijsen's *Citizenship and the Ethics of Care*, for instance, 'documents a search for ways of placing care within conceptions of democratic citizenship' (1998: 2). In a subsequent critique of the 'third way', she argues that 'the relationship between rights, obligation and responsibility cannot be theorized in an adequate manner without taking care into account in the fullest possible manner' (2000: 6). Knijn and Kremer (1997) have argued for the right to time to care and to receive care as part of an inclusive citizenship agenda.

This is a central issue for the Government's welfare reform strategy that has not been properly addressed. It also raises the wider question of what kind of support should be provided in order to guarantee the financial security of those unable to undertake paid work for whatever reason.

The 'welfare' reform agenda.

In theory, support for those unable to take paid work is covered by the central principle guiding the Green Paper on welfare reform, cited above: 'work for those who can; security for those who cannot'. In practice, a number of question marks remain over the Government's strategy to ensure 'security for those who cannot' undertake paid work. The Green Paper's vision is of 'Welfare 2020', built on 'three core values of work, security and opportunity' (DSS 1998: 79). 'At the heart of the modern welfare state', it declares, 'will be a new contract between the citizen and the Government based on responsibilities and rights' (DSS, 1998: 80), although, in line with the philosophy outlined earlier, the emphasis is more on the former than the latter. Having listed the duties of government and of the individual, the 'new welfare contract' sets out as a 'duty of us all'

> to help all individuals and families to realise their full potential and live a dignified life, by promoting economic independence through work, by relieving poverty where it cannot be prevented and by *building a strong and cohesive society where rights are matched by responsibilities.*
>
> (DSS 1998: 80, emphasis added)

In his Foreword, Blair describes the essence of the strategy as a 'third way', which is spelt out in the Green Paper in terms of the welfare state facing 'a choice of futures'. On the one side is 'a privatised future' with a residual safety-net for the poorest, which is rejected as divisive. On the other, is a status quo supported by those who 'believe that poverty is relieved exclusively by cash hand outs'. This too is rejected in favour of the third way: 'a modern form of welfare that believes in empowerment not dependency' (DSS 1998: 19).

Paid work is the route to empowerment, through an *active* welfare state, while improving benefit levels is equated with a *passive* welfare state which encourages dependency. The research evidence, which suggests that inadequate benefits for those out of work could undermine the Government's educational and welfare to work policies (summarized in Lister 1998), is discounted. Of particular significance here is social security's potential role in helping people to take risks. As Giddens (1998: 116) observes, 'deciding to go to work and give up benefits' is a 'risk-infused' action. There is evidence to suggest that, without the protection of a reasonable safety net, benefit claimants are less likely to be willing to take the risk of a job in a labour market, which offers many of the workless only temporary, part-time, self-employed or low skill jobs (McLaughlin 1994). Likewise, one study found that the greater the hardship experienced by lone mothers, the less likely they are to move into employment (Bryson *et al.* 1997: 29). It is through such evidence, contrasted with the reluctance to improve benefit levels for fear of encouraging 'dependency', that the false dichotomy between 'active' and 'passive' welfare is revealed most sharply.

In fact, a few carefully targeted benefit increases have been announced for groups who cannot be expected to seek work (poorer pensioners and severely disabled people). This reflects a distinction made by New Labour, influenced by the American David Ellwood, between those who are expected to look to the labour market for support and those who are not (Deacon 2000). Perhaps surprisingly, given that children's benefits are channelled through their parents, the improvements have included a 72 per cent phased increase in the income support rates for under-11 year olds. The first phase in the 1998 Budget can be understood as an attempt to take the sting out of the unpopular cuts in lone parents' benefits announced earlier. The second phase, in contrast, was mentioned in the 1999 Budget speech only in a cryptic aside. By focusing on children, the Government is able to do what it said it would not do, but is doing it so quietly that it does not always get credit for it.

More consistent with the New Labour philosophy is the doubling of the maternity grant to £200 (increased to £300 in 2000), but 'in return for parents meeting their responsibilities', i.e. the grant will be conditional on attendance at child health check ups. This is a completely new departure in British social security policy but a long-established practice in France, where children and their physical well-being have traditionally been a public concern.

For all the improvements that have been made, the more general case for a comprehensive review of the adequacy of benefit levels for those not in work has not been conceded, despite the fact that there has been no such public, official, review since the levels proposed by Beveridge.

What the Third Way in welfare reform means for the *structure* of social security is still ambiguous. The Green Paper's rejection of a residual safety net model and espousal of a welfare state 'from which we all benefit' (although it is not always clear when the term 'welfare state' is being used in its broad sense or in the narrower sense of social security) points to a more institutional model of social security. Yet, the lack of any commitment to reduce the scope of means-testing and the emphasis on private forms of provision (as part of a more general emphasis on 'partnership' between public and private sectors) do indicate a more limited two-tier model of provision, rather than one which gives the state a central role in ensuring the financial security of all its citizens.

The future of national insurance, widely viewed as the hallmark of the Beveridge model of social citizenship, has not been addressed explicitly either in the Green Paper or subsequently apart from the occasional opaque mention. Yet social insurance can be seen as promoting many of the Government's own principles and objectives including the notion of a welfare contract, the centrality of paid work and the provision of security in the face of risk (Bennett 1999).

One of the main criticisms of the current national insurance scheme is that it no longer adequately provides security to help people cope with the changing nature of economic and social risk. This was addressed by the Commission on Social Justice in the context of its belief that 'far from making the welfare state redundant, social and economic change creates a new and even more vital need for the security which the welfare state was designed to provide' (1994: 222).[5] The Commission put forward proposals for a modernized, more inclusive social insurance system, and one which is better attuned to the position and needs of many women. These proposals have been, more or less, ignored by the Government. While there have been some policy initiatives consistent with the Commission's position, others, which contribute to the drift towards greater reliance on means-testing and private provision, will weaken women's position.

The Government is disinclined to debate the shape of the social security system's underlying architecture. Alistair Darling, the Social Security Secretary, regards such debates as 'arid' and 'dogmatic'. He is more interested in what is 'cost-effective' and in 'outcomes' (DSS 1999; Hansard 1999). Likewise, Blair used his

Beveridge lecture to stress that in the mix of 'universal and targeted help', 'the one is not "superior" or "more principled" than the other' (Blair 1999: 13). The result is that, as Darling pursues his 'benefit by benefit' review, there is a danger that the shift under the Conservatives away from a social insurance based social security system towards a means-tested based one, is being continued by default. The Government has not attempted to encourage public debate about the appropriate balance between the different kinds of benefits – contributory, means-tested and contingency. Yet, its own Social Security Advisory Committee has warned of the consequences of the current direction of policy. Having identified 'the balance between the maintenance of the contributory principle and the targeting of benefits to those perceived as in greatest need' as an issue of 'significant concern', it suggests that current policy, in particular the changes to incapacity benefit and widows' benefits, signal a shift 'further towards targeted benefits . . . and . . . away from the social insurance principle'. The Committee believes

> that there is merit in the assertions of some commentators that the maintenance of a contributory element within the benefits structure means that all citizens, however well able they may be to provide for themselves, have a stake in that structure as potential recipients of benefit. Without this, the national insurance contribution may become seen by the affluent simply as a synonym for direct taxation. At the same time the principle of inclusive social insurance can be said to play a part in engendering social solidarity and cohesion.
> (Social Security Advisory Committee 1999: paras 7, 10 and 8)

David Piachaud reaches a similar conclusion in an analysis of the Government's pensions strategy, suggesting that 'the integrity of the social insurance system will steadily diminish' (1999a: 5). As a result, he warns, 'Britain risks being the only major OECD country without a secure social insurance foundation to tackle poverty' (1999b: 159). Going even further, Nicholas Timmins, Public Policy Editor of the *Financial Times*, has declared that 'national insurance is dead. . . . Government ministers know they are accelerating its destruction, but do not want to talk about it much' (22 November 1999). *The Economist* has declared approvingly that 'Tony Blair's Government has crossed the Rubicon from . . . the left bank of welfare-for-all to the right bank of means testing' (6 March 1999). Even if possibly something of an overstatement (given, for example, counter-indications such as the increases in the real value of child benefit), these observations act as a hazard warning. Instead of a 'Third Way' in social security reform, we may be moving further down the road towards the very model rejected in the Green Paper, that of a residual poverty relief social security system typical of liberal regimes such as the USA, even if, as argued by Howard Glennerster (1999), the specific policy lane is different from that adopted in the USA. This takes us further away from more institutionalized Continental European models, which are themselves also under pressure (Clasen 1997; Cox 1998).

Some have suggested that the main impetus for the crossing of the benefits Rubicon comes from the Treasury, although Gordon Brown's enthusiasm for child benefit is not totally consistent with that. Interestingly, the Treasury is playing an increasingly proactive role in the development of social policy, reflecting Brown's own interest. Treasury intervention is focused on children in particular. Examples include the Treasury-inspired Sure Start scheme and working families tax credit (WFTC), to be subsumed, in turn, into a new integrated child credit (ICC). The latter will, it is claimed, provide a single, seamless income-related system of support for children, paid to the main carer (in acknowledgement of the criticisms of the gendered effects of paying the WFTC mainly through the wage packet, see Goode *et al*. 1998). The ICC will be complemented by an employment credit for low paid working adults, with suggestions that the long term goal is a fully integrated tax-benefit system.

For all its proactive social policy stance and despite the partial rehabilitation of public expenditure as a positive tool of Government, reflected in particular in a significant increase in health spending announced in 2000, the Treasury continues to operate within the low tax, limited public spending paradigm espoused by the Thatcher Government. In this way, New Labour has deliberately distanced itself from 'Old Labour's 'tax and spend' policies (although, it was, in fact, the 1974–79 Labour Government that started the retreat from public spending in the face of demands from the IMF).

In search of the 'Big Idea'

The use of the term New Labour acts as a deliberate, constant reminder that this is not the Labour Party of old. The promotion of New Labour is buttressed by a discourse of modernization and change, which runs through all its policy documents and political statements. It is a discourse that brooks no opposition. It is also one which creates a sense of inevitability, denying the choices involved in *how* politics responds to economic and social change (Finlayson 1998; Hay 1998).

The Third Way represents New Labour's response to change. Blair has described it as 'an attempt to say there's a principled position which is also entirely sensible, and it is about taking the values of the left – social justice, solidarity, community, democracy, liberty – and recasting them and reshaping them for the new world' (*The Guardian*, 15 May 1998). A key example given by Blair of Third Way policies is 'the embracing of globalisation as inevitable and also as desirable' so that competitiveness in this global market is combined with 'active' labour market and education and training policies 'to equip people for that' (ibid.).

The exact location of the Third Way, in terms of its political geography, remains unclear. In the face of initial criticisms of the Third Way's bias to the right, both Blair (1998a) and Giddens (1998) have appeared to be using the compass of a modernized social democracy, committed to social justice, in order to fix the Third Way's bearings. Nevertheless, the move 'beyond left and right' has been denounced as implying that 'we live in a society which is no longer structured by social division' (Mouffe 1998: 13). Here, a genuine dichotomy is glossed over while, at the same time, the diversity of previous Left and Right positions is ignored. In particular, all pre-New Labour thinking on the centre-left is lumped together as 'Old' and therefore by implication irrelevant to these new times. This writes out of political and intellectual history a body of political thinking that goes under various rubrics but would include the notions of 'radical democracy' and 'critical social policy'. Not only are they ignored in the distorted image of existing Left thinking that is presented, but, even more importantly, their ideas do not appear to be informing in any systematic or fundamental way the construction of the Third Way alternative to it.

In particular, there has been only limited engagement with attempts to forge a citizenship 'politics of difference' or 'recognition', especially as vocalized through the demands of various 'grassroots' groups and social movements not simply for equality but also to have their differences respected and their particular needs acknowledged. In the context of constitutional reform and the challenge of Scottish nationalism, both Blair and Brown have, however, emphasized the diversity of the UK's peoples, at a rhetorical level at least. Indeed, the latter has written of his vision of a Britain where unity springs from 'celebrating diversity, in other words a multicultural, multi-ethnic and multinational Britain' which will require a move from a 'Britain of subjects to a modern pluralist democracy – the Britain of citizens'. This, he argued, will require both constitutional change and 'unifying ideas of citizenship' (*The Guardian*, 12 November 1998).[6]

A politics of difference or recognition has never been adequately represented through the formal political system. Highly pertinent, therefore, is another New Labour ideal of an 'inclusive politics'. In an *Observer* interview with Roy Hattersley, Blair seemed to be interpreting an inclusive Left politics as one which appealed to the aspirational, the successful and the powerful (3 May 1998). This may make narrow electoral sense, but a wider conception of politics suggests that it is the relatively power*less* rather than the power*ful* that an 'inclusive politics' should be trying to reach.

The formal political system tends to exclude minority ethnic groups, disabled people, people in poverty and, despite the breakthrough in the last general election, women. New Labour has made a concerted attempt to feminize its image. The existence of a number of 'out' gay and lesbian Members of Parliament, including some ministers, suggests a greater openness around sexuality. But it is still a very white government and there have been a number of criticisms of the failure to reflect the country's multi-ethnic composition in political and quasi-political appointments (Alibhai Brown 1999).

There are some attempts now to open up the political system through a variety of means, reflecting what Blair calls the Third Way's 'democratic impulse' which, he states, 'needs to be strengthened by finding new ways to enable citizens to share in decision-making that affects them' (Blair 1998a: 15). Citizens' juries, a 'listening to women initiative' from the Women's Unit (an Old Labour policy commitment which Blair did not feel able to jettison), a 'race relations forum', a 'listening to older people' initiative and a 'people's panel' to elicit views on public services are among the devices to further this goal.

However, despite the welfare reform Green Paper's evocation of the image of 'the demanding sceptical citizen-consumer', there is no discussion of extending to the social security system the principles of user-involvement beginning to be developed in welfare services as 'the site for the pursuit of active citizenship' by 'citizen-consumers' (Williams, 1999: 683). As Robert Walker has observed,

> there is scope for user involvement not only in the delivery of services but also in the planning, development, monitoring, evaluation and implementation of policy. Experience in other sectors, most noticeably social services, suggests that this can promote personal growth and citizenship, combat stigma, engender better communications and enhance the quality of decision-making.
>
> (Walker 1998: 81)

Blair's observation, in the Government's first Annual Report, that 'in all walks of life people act as consumers and not just citizens' suggests that it is the consumer rather than the citizen who represents the ideal New Labour welfare subject (Blair 1998b: 6).

Likewise, hitherto little or no effort has been made to involve as citizens those marginalized by poverty whose voices are rarely heard in public debates about poverty and welfare reform. The political exclusion of those in poverty has intensified alongside their social and economic exclusion. There is a growing demand among some activists and academics that anti-poverty debates and action should be participatory, involving as full, active, citizens those who stand to be affected. This would be in line with the UN Copenhagen Declaration to which the UK is a signatory.

Conclusion

It is still difficult to reach definitive conclusions as to the nature of the route being mapped out as a Third Way for 'welfare' reform. Cutting through the thickets of rhetoric to discern the actual path is not always easy, particularly when the two seem to be pointing in different directions. It is this dissonance between New Labour's rhetoric and the reality of certain policies, and between competing rhetorics, which will be highlighted by way of a conclusion. It is a dissonance which operates in more than one direction and in a number of ways.

First, despite the continued espousal of the rhetoric of social justice, it is, arguably, primarily a social cohesion model of social inclusion to which New Labour subscribes. While the two are not necessarily incompatible, the promotion of a narrow social cohesion model, which ignores wider inequalities of resources and power, runs the risk of becoming detached from principles of social justice, for all New Labour's continued rhetorical commitment to them. Its rejection of greater equality as an overall objective raises serious questions about its ability to meet the historic goal of the eradication of child poverty in two decades (made by Blair in his 1999 Beveridge Lecture) and to end social exclusion in the face of entrenched inequalities of income, wealth and power.

Second, Blair (1999: 12) also used his Beveridge Lecture to contrast the popularity of the Beveridge welfare state with its unpopularity today, as it has become 'associated with fraud, abuse, laziness, a dependency culture, social irresponsibility encouraged by welfare dependency'. He rightly stressed the need to make the system popular again, if taxpayers are to be persuaded to fund it. Yet, arguably his own Government's negative language about welfare, with its talk of a 'dependency culture' and 'fraudsters', might be counter-productive to this task. The potential impact of such language on how benefit claimants are seen by the wider society, and also on how they see themselves, should not be underestimated.

Third, behind this negative language and the tough talk of work not benefits, some limited improvements in benefits for those not in work, which do not really fit the New Labour template, are quietly being put in place. It is not clear to what extent these reflect tensions in the New Labour project and to what extent they represent a clear political strategy of (strictly limited) redistribution by stealth, carried out in such a way as not to frighten Middle England *Daily Mail* readers. Either way, by focusing on children, the Government can harness its rhetoric of opportunity to redistribute resources to a group more likely to evoke public sympathy. Of course, this redistribution has to be channelled through their parents. So, for instance, Brown has contrasted old forms of redistribution based on 'something for nothing' with redistribution based on 'people exercising responsibilities' to work and, significantly here, to bring up their children (*Today Programme*, BBC Radio 4, 29 March 1999).

What we are perhaps seeing is 'redistribution with a purpose' i.e. not redistribution for its own sake in the name of greater equality but redistribution to promote RIO. In many ways this is a very positive development. A bit of old-fashioned redistribution to a group, particularly vulnerable to poverty and its effects, is being carried out in the name of opportunity and responsibility. This perhaps signals implicit acknowledgement of earlier criticisms of New Labour's work-biased construction of citizenship responsibilities and that genuine equality of opportunity requires some redistribution of resources as well as of endowments. Yet, as argued earlier, redistribution by stealth can only go so far. Moreover, very welcome and appropriate as the priority being given to children is, in the long run the individual needs of their parents and of other adults cannot be ignored.

Finally, there is something of a tension between the rhetoric of 'radical welfare reform' and the more prosaic and pragmatic 'what works' approach emphasized by Darling, though the two are bound together by the discourse of modernization. As Powell and Hewitt (1998) observe, by focusing public discussion on to more technical issues of cost-effectiveness, attention is diverted from important issues of principle. Darling, in particular, is impatient with suggestions that the direction of reform is away from more Continental European models towards a more US-type poverty relief model. Yet, the sum effect of a series of pragmatic steps could be a significant shift in the overall model of social security, without adequate public debate about the principles at stake. As Esping-Andersen's welfare regime analysis (1990) underlines, this has implications for the overall fabric of social relations and social citizenship. As means-tested and private forms of provision play a more dominant role, it is likely to spell greater financial insecurity for many and lead to a more fractured model of social citizenship.

Notes

1 This chapter is based on a paper given at the Equality and Democratic State Conference, Vancouver (November 1998) which is being published in E. Broadbent (forthcoming) *Equality and the Democratic State*, University of Toronto Press. A longer version is being published in C. Hay (ed.) (2001) *British Politics Today*, Polity.

2 The possibility of using social security policy to combat anti-social behaviour has been raised in the 2000 Housing Green Paper. This floats the idea of reducing housing benefit and other housing-related payments 'to encourage responsible behaviour' amongst 'unruly tenants' (DETR 2000: paras. 5.47 & 5.46).

3 Working families tax credit replaced family credit as the main source of meanstested support for low income working families. It is considerably more generous than the family credit and incorporates a child care credit. It was designed to be paid through the wage-packet, but see the discussion later.

4 Under considerable pressure the Government has now agreed to review the question of paid parental leave as part of a wider review of maternity and parental leave provisions.

5 The Commission on Social Justice was set up by the late John Smith, Leader of the Labour Opposition, as an independent body 'to develop a practical vision of economic and social reform for the twenty-first Century'.

6 It was hoped that the report on the Stephen Lawrence Inquiry would provide the catalyst to turn some of this rhetoric into serious action for change across the board. There has, indeed, been progress on some fronts but the progress is not consistent. In particular, the Government's punitive approach to asylum-seekers, from whom all rights to social security benefits as such have been removed, does not exactly send out a signal of multi-ethnic inclusive citizenship.

References

Alibhai Brown, Y. (1999) *True Colours. Public Attitudes to Multiculturalism and the role of government*, London: Institute for Public Policy Research.

Beer, S. (1998) 'The roots of New Labour. Liberalism rediscovered', *The Economist*, 7 February: 23–5.

Bennett, F. (1999) Social Security Committee Oral Evidence, HC485–IV, 14.7.99.

Bennett, F. and Walker, R. (1998) *Working with Work. An initial assessment of welfare to work*, York: Joseph Rowntree Foundation.

Blair, T. (1995) 'The rights we enjoy reflect the duties we owe', Spectator Lecture, London, 22 March.

—— (1998a) *The Third Way. New Politics for the New Century*, London: Fabian Society.

—— (1998b) 'The Government's strategy', *The Government's Annual Report 97/98*, London: HMSO.

—— (1999) Beveridge Lecture, Toynbee Hall, London, 18 March, reproduced in R. Walker (1999) *Ending Child Poverty. Popular Welfare for the 21st Century?* Bristol: Policy Press.

Bryson, A., Ford, R. and White, M. (1997) *Making Work Pay: Lone Mothers, Employment and Well-being*, York: Joseph Rowntree Foundation.

Clasen, J. (ed.) (1997) *Social Insurance in Europe*, Bristol: The Policy Press.

Commission on Social Justice (1994) *Social Justice: Strategies for National Renewal*, London: Vintage.

Cox, R.H. (1998) 'The consequences of welfare reform: how conceptions of social rights are changing', *Journal of Social Policy* 21(1): 1–16.

Deacon, A. (1997) '"Welfare to work": options and issues', in M. May, E. Brunsdon and G. Craig (eds) *Social Policy Review 9*, London: Social Policy Association.

—— (2000) 'Learning from the US? The influence of American ideas upon "new labour" thinking on welfare reform', *Policy & Politics* 28(1): 5–18.

DETR (Department of Environment, Transport and Regions) (2000) *Quality and Choice: A Decent Home for All: The Housing Green Paper*, London: DETR.

Driver, S. and Martell, L. (1998) *New Labour. Politics after Thatcherism*, Cambridge: Polity Press.

DSS (1998) *New Ambitions for Our Country: A New Contract for Welfare*, London: HMSO.

—— (1999) 'Means Testing: The History', unpublished note for meeting with Social Security Consortium.

Duncan, S. and Edwards, R. (1999) *Lone Mothers, Paid Work and Gendered Moral Rationalities*, Basingstoke: Macmillan.

Esping-Andersen, G. (1990) *The Three Worlds of Welfare Capitalism*, Cambridge: Polity.

Finlayson, A. (1998) 'Tony Blair and the jargon of modernisation', *Soundings* 10: 11–27.

Fitzpatrick, T. (1998) 'The rise of market collectivism', in E. Brunsdon, H. Dean and R. Woods (eds) *Social Policy Review 10*, London: Social Policy Association.

Ford, R. (1996) *Childcare in the Balance*, London: Policy Studies Institute.

Fraser, N. (1997) *Justice Interruptus*, New York and London: Routledge.

Freeden, M. (1999) 'The ideology of New Labour', *Political Quarterly* 70(1): 42–51.

Giddens, A. (1998) *The Third Way. The Renewal of Social Democracy*, Cambridge: Polity Press.

Glennerster, H. (1999) 'A third way?' in H. Dean and R. Woods (eds) (1999) *Social Policy Review 11*, Luton: Social Policy Association.

Goode, J., Callender, C. and Lister, R. (1998) *Purse or Wallet? Gender Inequalities and Income Distribution within Families on Benefits*, London: Policy Studies Institute.

Hansard (1999) 19 November, col. 309.

Hay, C. (1998) 'Globalisation, welfare retrenchment and the "logic of no alternative"; why second-best won't do', *Journal of Social Policy* 27(4): 525–32.

Knijn, T. and Kremer, M. (1997) 'Gender and the caring dimension of welfare states: towards inclusive citizenship', *Social Politics*, 4(3): 328–61.

Levitas, R. (1998) *The Inclusive Society? Social Exclusion and New Labour*, Basingstoke: Macmillan.

Lister, R. (1996) 'In search of the "underclass"', in R. Lister (ed.) *Charles Murray and the Underclass. The Developing Debate*, London: Institute of Economic Affairs in association with *The Sunday Times*.

—— (1997) *Citizenship: Feminist Perspectives*, Basingstoke: Macmillan.

—— (1998) 'Fighting social exclusion . . . with one hand tied behind our back', *New Economy*, 5(1): 14–18.

—— (1999) 'What welfare provisions do women need to become full citizens?', in S. Walby (ed.) *New Agendas for Women*, Basingstoke: Macmillan.

McLaughlin, E. (1994) *Flexibility in Work and Benefits*, London: Institute for Public Policy Research.

Mouffe, C. (1998) 'The radical centre: A politics without adversary', *Soundings* 9: 11–23.

Piachaud, D. (1999a) 'Security for old age?' *Benefits* 26: 1–6.

—— (1999b) 'Progress on poverty', *New Economy* 6(3): 154–60.

Powell, M. and Hewitt, M. (1998) 'The end of the welfare state?' *Social Policy & Administration*, 32(1): 1–13.

Sevenhuijsen, S. (1998) *Citizenship and the Ethics of Care*, London and New York: Routledge.

—— (2000) 'Caring in the third way: the relation between obligation, responsibility and care in *Third Way* discourse', *Critical Social Policy* 20(1): 5–37.

Social Security Advisory Committee (1999), *Twelfth Report*, May 1997–March 1999, London: HMSO.

Turock, I. and Edge, N. (1999) *The Jobs Gap in Britain's Cities: Employment Loss and Labour Market Consequences*, Bristol: The Policy Press.

Turok, I. and Webster, D. (1998) 'The New Deal: Jeopardised by the geography of unemployment?', *Local Economy* 13: 309–28.

Walker, R. (1998) 'Promoting positive welfare', *New Economy*, 5(2): 77–82.

Williams, F. (1999) 'Good enough principles for welfare', *Journal of Social Policy*, 28(4): 667–87.

Chapter 8

Managing the risk
of unemployment
Is welfare restructuring undermining support for social security?

David Abbott and Deborah Quilgars

Introduction

The present Government is increasingly placing the emphasis on paid work as offering the route out of poverty for those households that have been reliant on benefits following unemployment, lone parenthood or, in some cases, disability. There is no doubt that employment, for the vast majority of households in Britain, is seen as both a desirable, as well as an economically beneficial state. This chapter does not refute this, rather it seeks to explore what government policy in this area might really mean for individuals and households, particularly low income ones, with the backdrop of changing labour markets and welfare re-structuring. Flexibilization of labour, bringing higher levels of insecurity, now exists alongside a shrinking safety net for the unemployed, with the Government placing increased responsibilities on families to plan for their own welfare. Using data from in-depth interviews from a major research study,[1] this chapter looks at how respondents living with quite high degrees of job insecurity, often living on the edge of benefits, manage in this new risk economy.

The chapter begins with a discussion of the shifting labour and welfare markets in Britain, charting in more detail how increasing risks of unemployment have occurred at the same time as significant reductions in safety net provision. The assumptions on which these policies have been pursued are questioned. In light of these changes, the chapter then examines respondents' experiences and views in two main areas: first, the way people, particularly those most constrained by income, plan for the future, including any risk of unemployment they may perceive; and second, the welfare views of the respondents: who do they believe should support people who are unemployed? The chapter highlights the considerable structural barriers to planning amongst lower income households and how a 'hierarchy' of planning means that unemployment risks are amongst the last to be addressed at an individual level. An examination of welfare views reveals some potentially far-reaching assumptions and beliefs about collective state insurance and its role in supporting unemployed people. The chapter ends by reflecting more broadly on the implications of shifts in welfare policy, and possibly in welfare views: is welfare restructuring, within a context of increased flexibilization of the workforce, undermining the support for social security? And if it is, what are the implications for those people in low paid work?

Shifting ground: increasing risk, reducing security

The way that European nation states have, in varying ways, moved to create more flexible labour markets in response to the powers of globalization has been discussed in detail elsewhere (Esping-Anderson 1996). In Britain, a neo-liberal approach to labour policy has involved widespread deregulation to produce an essentially low wage economy, with few employment rights but greater labour mobility (movement of workers between jobs). Whilst most of the changes were presided over by a Conservative administration (especially the curtailment of trade union powers, as well as the reduction of statutory redundancy rights in 1993), and the incoming Labour Government has established some minimum standards (most obviously through introducing a minimum wage in 1999), the Labour Government has repeatedly stated its commitment to a flexible labour market (HM Treasury 1997; Department of Trade and Industry 1998).

There is now substantial evidence of increased employment risk and the existence of, at least in part, a flexible labour market in Britain. Whilst a majority of economically active heads of household were still in full-time permanent employment in 1997/98, the increase in part-time work and self-employment (Lindley and Wilson, 1998), means that approximately a third of heads of households now occupy more 'risky' labour market positions (self-employment, part-time work, temporary work and unemployment) (Labour Force Survey, reported in Quilgars and Abbott 2000). In addition, a recent Omnibus survey of individuals showed that of those currently in employment (or self-employment in the last 5 years) 30 per cent had experienced at least one spell of unemployment in the last five years (Cebulla et al. 1998). However, these headline figures hide the unequal distribution of risky jobs between households and different groups in the population, and within households themselves. For example, the same data showed that half of households renting accommodation had a head of household in a risky labour market position compared to only a quarter of owner occupiers. The UK Labour Force Survey data for Autumn 1997 also show that unemployment rates were six times as great for unskilled workers, at 12 per cent, compared to a low of 2 per cent for professionals (Cebulla et al. 1998).

At the same time as employment has been becoming more risky, subsequent governments' long-term objective of transferring some of the state's post-war traditional areas of welfare responsibility to the individual householder has progressed. Whilst the state still provides the main 'safety net' for households facing unemployment, welfare provision in this area has been eroded by a number of measures. On the contributory side of benefits, from 1996 unemployment benefit calculated from National Insurance contributions was cut from 12 months to 6 months. Meanstested benefits were also reduced for home owners. New owner occupiers taking out a mortgage since October 1995, who subsequently have difficulties in meeting payments, now face a nine month qualifying period for assistance with interest payments through the income support system (ISMI). The recent Housing Green Paper (DETR 2000), whilst outlining a welcome extension of linking arrangements (the amount of time people can work for, when coming off benefits, before they have to re-qualify for benefits again should that employment cease) from 13 to 52 weeks, also raises the possibility of extending the waiting period for ISMI to 14 months at some point in the future. This measure, along with a few other changes, would be

> designed to link in better with private insurance (MPPI), encouraging homeowners to make increased provision for unforeseen circumstances, reducing the burden on the state, and rewarding responsible behaviour.
>
> (DETR 2000: 39)

Two major assumptions underlie a government policy which seeks to shift the burden of responsibility and cost from the state to individual households to cover the increased risks associated with more flexible labour markets. These assumptions, however, can be shown to be erroneous, or at the very least, problematic.

First, there is an assumption that private insurance markets can efficiently and effectively provide an adequate safety net against the effects of unemployment. Evidence suggests that whilst private insurance may be able to insure some relatively straightforward risks associated with employment (for example, the risk of redundancy), there are many areas that the private market finds harder to cover (for example, people with problematic health and/or employment profiles), and some areas which are uninsurable (such as unemployment as a result of caring responsibilities or relationship breakdown). Most importantly, this often means that those in the most risky labour market situations, those that need the protection the most, are those who are least likely to be able to protect themselves. For example, those in the riskier labour market positions are more likely to have their claim for MPPI rejected (Kempson *et al.* 1999). Whilst a social policy may be designed to help those in greatest need, insurance companies are, in contrast, concerned with avoiding adverse selection, that is avoiding a situation where those who represent the worst risk are the most likely to insure against that risk.

Second, changes in public policy have been made with implicit assumptions about how individuals will respond to unemployment risk. There has been an assumption that people will perceive such risks, and further that they will be willing, and able, to act on this perceived risk. It is therefore presumed that people will make a rational decision to take out private insurance; and those who do not do so are likely to be acting irresponsibly. A separate paper, based on the same research study reported here (Quilgars and Abbott 2000), showed that whilst those in paid employment are acutely aware of the general trend towards greater job insecurity, there is no necessary correlation between their own feelings of (in)security and objective assessments of their labour market position. Individuals perceive and assess unemployment risk in a much more complex way than is implicitly presumed within policy, taking account of a range of social, economic and personal factors, as well as labour market position. Questions placed on the British Household Panel Survey (waves 1996/7 and 1997/8) for the same study also showed that two in three of those who became unemployed during that year failed to foresee that event (Cebulla and Ford 2000).

It may be asserted that policy is seriously flawed if it presumes that people will perceive risks in the labour market according to some economic calculation of risk; assessments made by families are much more complex and subtle (Ford 1999). This assumption, combined with one which presumes that private insurance can effectively provide protection against the effects of unemployment, underlies much of present policy yet evidence suggests that this leaves significant sections of the population inadequately protected against the risk of unemployment.

The research study

In 1996, a three year study was funded by the main social sciences funding body in the UK, the Economic and Social Research Council, as part of their Risk and Human Behaviour Programme, to explore and document families' perceptions of, and responses to, the risk of unemployment. The study combined both quantitative and qualitative methodologies, including a comparison of subjective perceptions of risks with actuarial risk. This chapter concentrates on the qualitative interviews carried out with employed respondents.

In 1997 and 1998, 90 semi-structured, one-to-one interviews were conducted with members of 50 households in two local authority areas of England: Leicester, an ethnically diverse, urban area, with a varied labour market with both large service and industry sectors; and Selby, North Yorkshire, a small town, set in a rural hinterland, with a less varied labour market. Both areas, however, had seen changes in the structure of the local labour market with the decline of the textile and coal mining industries, in Leicester and Selby respectively. The research sought to interview individuals from different socio-economic groups, within different household structures and housing tenures. Twenty couples with children, 20 couples without children and 10 lone parents were interviewed. There was an even split between owners and renters and between socio-economic groups AB (professional/ managerial/ technical occupations), C1/ C2 (non-manual and manual skilled trades) and D (semi-skilled/ unskilled). All respondents in Selby were of a white ethnic origin; five of the twenty-five households interviewed in Leicester included respondents from ethnic minorities. Interviews were included with people of all working ages, although the very young (under 25) were under-represented.

In examining responses to the risk of unemployment, this chapter focuses primarily on the strategies of those who in many ways faced the greatest challenge to providing security for themselves and their families: those at the margins of work and benefits and most constrained by lack of income (the Ds). However, the chapter also makes comparisons between different socio-economic groups, particularly in considering welfare views.

Planning for unemployment: constraints and priorities

The study included interviews with adults in 19 households (34 interviews) where the main earner was in an unskilled/semi-skilled occupation, and therefore classified as socio-economic group D. Two thirds of these households were renting accommodation; a third buying their house. All but one household included children; and six households consisted of lone mothers and their children. Within the couple households, all the male partners, with one exception, were in paid employment, whilst half of the female partners were looking after the home. All the lone mothers were in paid work. In general, male employment was characterized by greater degrees of self-perceived insecurity than female employment. In particular, women tended to feel more work secure (that is, they felt they would be able to secure another similar job should they lose their present one) than men who felt that they might face periods of unemployment if they lost their present job.

Financial household planning, both generally, and specifically for the possibility of future unemployment, was heavily constrained by family income. However, this did not mean that people did not plan; rather it meant they planned in different ways. Most people were acutely aware of the resources available to them and how they had to be closely managed to meet the household's needs. Planning, first and foremost, centred around planning to manage and to meet necessities. This could involve highly structured approaches to planning. One household literally had different boxes for the different areas of expenditure and income would be split between these boxes, for example, for the mortgage, car tax, children's uniforms as well as a holiday fund. Another household drew up weekly lists of expenditure before allocating income. One mother looking after the home said:

> We have to plan for things like buying new school uniforms . . . so in the summer holidays I'm going to have to buy one thing a week. Do you see what I mean? . . . so planning ahead you have to plan like that, but that's for the kids. But for yourself you don't. Its just a waste of time. You take it day by day. It's the best way and then you're not going to feel so let down if something goes wrong.

Most respondents focused on planning to manage over the short term, as opposed to planning to save for the longer term which was seen as problematic. Some felt it was not possible at all, explaining how they managed almost 'hand to mouth'. Most could however undertake modest savings, but this was usually reserved for savings for specific items or occasions, like a family holiday or Xmas. As well as planning to save over the long term being problematic, very few people saved simply for the sake of saving. A part-time chambermaid stated: 'We can't afford to put money aside for no reason, really.'

When people tried to save more generally, they explained how such reserves usually got used for an unexpected expenditure. Quite a few families felt that 'something always comes up', or that planning 'never works': 'We can't really make plans for the future. We try to, but every week something different crops up, so that spoils it.' Any planning of a longer term nature had to be subject to revision over time. Three respondents had had to freeze pensions on account of increased expenditure (with most not having pensions), and others described cashing in insurance policies or savings plans. A female shop assistant, with a taxi driver partner, explained:

> I think of the future constantly, but the amount that you actually . . . you know
> . . . we could never guarantee that we'd have the money every week. I mean
> he has been in pensions schemes before, but not for any length of time.

Where people were managing to save on a regular basis, the savings were modest, for example one family had two small insurance policies of £3 a week. In consequence this meant the expected benefits of such policies would also be modest in time. The biggest planning for some involved the buying of their home which they saw as planning for the future. Quite a few people stressed the importance of having opportunities for flexible planning and being able to take breaks from saving when resources were tight. However, it was perceived that financial services were becoming less rather than more flexible. A cavity wall insulator said:

> Insurances for accidents and that – we just can't afford it every week. I mean
> if someone came round and knocked on your door and it were like £10 a week,
> I'd maybe, you know, if he came round on a Friday at 6 o'clock and
> said, 'right, where's your money', I'd pay it and then that's it, done. But there's
> not many companies what do that now, at all.

A hierarchy of planning clearly existed with planning to manage in the short term coming first, followed by planning for death, planning for retirement and illness, and sometimes planning for children's education, and only further down the list came planning for unemployment. Planning for death would seem to have been a very instinctive kind of financial planning. It was often what the respondents' parents had done in the past. Amongst those living on tight resources, very small amounts were put aside in life insurance policies. Where this was possible it contributed some peace of mind as if, however difficult it was to plan for life's potential problems like illness or unemployment, there was one thing that could be done which could make a tangible and positive benefit for family after death. The importance of planning for death bridged all the socio-economic groups. However, in spite of the desire to make planning for the event of death a priority, this was not always available to all. A couple of people felt they could not afford life insurances which they felt were a very important protection for their families. One lone mother, who worked part-time as a cleaner, explained:

> It's more important that I can buy food and gas and electric with that money other than life insurance, should the worse happen then it will be dealt with and they will find a way, and I might have to go in a pauper's grave or something, I'm not really bothered what they do after.

The majority of respondents identified financial planning as being important. Payment protection on loans and home shopping catalogues were usually seen as good value for money. Only a couple of people had other income protection policies such as mortgage payment protection insurance or critical illness insurance. Whilst some were sceptical of the benefits of insurance, a couple felt they would like more cover for the risk of unemployment but were unable to take it out due to existing health problems which would make them ineligible. Belief in and desire for planning could be in conflict with the need to spend scarce resources on enjoying a reasonable standard of family living, so that treating the children and having a social life was often seen as a higher priority than planning, given limited resources. One father explained: 'I'd rather us lot lived rather than try and prepare for my own future.' With respect to planning for unemployment, feeling optimistic about one's re-employability or agency in coping with unemployment meant that planning for unemployment was not always seen as essential.

In some contrast, financial planning for the future *per se* was a key feature of the majority of respondents in socio-economic group A/B. This was in addition, and often related, to occupational advantages over others which already represented a good measure of security – better redundancy packages, sick pay, occupational pensions, holiday pay, contracts, etc. A number of AB respondents had made careful, deliberate financial planning decisions weighing up the advantages and disadvantages of different forms of investments. Only occasionally did AB respondents say that saving for the future was not a priority, although even here insurances were important for respondents with children. However only a couple of people had specifically planned for the event of redundancy. Those who had not done this felt that their general planning was enough to protect them, given the security of their job, re-employability or likely redundancy packages.

C1 and C2 respondents tended to straddle the responses of people in socio-economic group AB and D. Their occupations were varied and in some ways, they felt the least secure, attempting to hold onto a reasonable standard of living. Money was much tighter than for AB respondents but it did give some scope for making decisions about money – whether to save, invest, or spend. Two full-time incomes however were usually a prerequisite to taking out insurances and saving plans. C2 respondents were often in a poorer position as, like the Ds, they did not often earn enough to save or pay into a pension. A number were financially worse off than a decade ago as their wages had not increased with standard of living costs.

The ability of D respondents to plan for the eventuality of unemployment was clearly limited by a lack of income and the precariousness of work. Yet, given the absence of private alternatives to them, social security might be seen as the main financial fallback in the event of no other work being found or whilst job search went on. But how do the people themselves, who live closer to the edges of work and social security, view benefits? Do they see it as an effective fallback in the event of unemployment? What role, if any, do state benefits play for ABs and Cs when they think about their financial security? And do views on welfare differ across these socio-economic groups?

Views on social security as a backstop to the risk of unemployment

The vast majority of respondents – across all socio-economic groups – felt that the state should provide some support to people who became unemployed. Whilst many thought the state should take the sole or major role, alongside this, there was also a good measure of support for more 'mixed provision', i.e. some combination of help from the state with some in built assumption that people will have some of their own resources to fall back on. Only a very small minority, predominately from higher income groups, felt that the major, or entire, onus should be on individuals making private provision for themselves. Nonetheless, as discussed below, welfare views, between and within socio-economic groups, were quite complex and raised questions about the likely future support for welfare in some quarters.

Many people talked about how those who had paid in to the system deserved to be supported, but that there was abuse of the system which needed to be curbed. There was an overwhelming discourse on deserving and undeserving claimants amongst all groups of respondents. This was sometimes associated with pejorative comments about certain sections of the population, particularly people from non-white backgrounds. One man in an AB bracket said there were too many handouts and not enough self reliance, yet despite a very high joint income, he and his wife fought hard to get their daughter Disability Living Allowance (DLA). He said:

> I had to fight for my daughter to get DLA but because she lived in a nice house, her mummy and daddy both worked, her mummy and daddy were both married, her mummy and daddy were white, dare I say it, her mummy and daddy were articulate, we had to fight, we didn't have a social worker helping us.

Often, the 'undeserving' were simply seen as those people who were perceived to be unwilling to work. One D respondent explained:

> I think it should be the state. You pay for it. We all pay for it, and employers pay for it. Well, if you're unemployed and it's through no fault of your own,

then yeah, you should be provided, but like these that just don't want a job
and they're not willing to go and get a job, then, I think they should try and
find some means of . . .

Fraud was mentioned in virtually every conversation about social security and
raised strong opinions. Here, another D householder said: 'There are so many fraud
cases . . . there must be thousands and thousands of people out there who claim off
social security and have got full-time jobs.' However, whilst most Ds and Cs felt
that the state should support genuine unemployed people, it was interesting to note
that some people did not see social security as an effective backstop to them in
the event of unemployment. When asked what people would do in the event of
being faced with unemployment, most people mentioned first that they would find
alternative work; any work. Relying on state provision was more often seen as the
last resort, both because of the level of income it would bring but also because
of negative experiences of being a claimant. However, most Ds, in particular,
accepted that they would ultimately be reliant on state benefits as other resources
such as savings were minimal. All the same, people felt that it would be very
difficult to make ends meet on present levels of social security; some mentioned
working on the side to supplement income.

The majority of Cs also saw a role for the state in providing benefits to families
facing unemployment. In particular, there was a group of Cs who clearly felt that
the state should provide as the system operated on a contributory basis and they
had paid in, and therefore deserved to be supported. A self-employed plumber
stated: 'They've got our money remember. We've earned the money, we've paid
the tax. I've paid them tax. Where's my tax going?' However, for many Cs,
arguments centred much more on the contributory nature of the system than the
behaviour of people on benefits, as it did with Ds. Thus, a few felt that only those
who had helped themselves and had contributed to the system, and/or made other
provision too, should benefit (with the exception of those who clearly could not,
such as older people and disabled people). A factory supervisor gave this account:

> It all depends, I think, on the individual, whether they've been willing to help
> themselves out beforehand . . . I think people should be taken on what they've
> done to try and help themselves . . . I suppose that's strong morals from my
> parents, because my parents have always been like that. You don't live off the
> state and you pay your way.

One self-employed manageress wondered why she was still paying National
Insurance given the small benefits likely to be derived if she became unemployed,
coupled with the fact of paying for a number of private insurances:

> And you'd wonder what was the point in paying the national insurance
> and all the taxes because you're coming down and down on what the benefits
> are that you are actually getting from it . . . if you become unemployed you're

going to pay your own money back in through the insurances that you've paid, then in general the money you're losing off your wages again it's just another insurance but that one you're not going to get anything back for, that's just your contribution to perhaps what other people are being able to get that haven't paid insurances or what have you. So that doesn't seem fair.

However, analysis of respondents' views revealed that some ABs, in particular, were beginning to feel that they might be losing out on a bargain which they had previously been happy to sign up to. In other words, they felt that they were increasingly subsidizing a system in which more and more benefits were being taken away from them. In the face of making private provision for themselves in the knowledge that social security benefits would not meet their standards of living in the event of unemployment, they were beginning to wonder what they got out of being in a relationship with the social security system. One AB man thought that this was acceptable as long as it did not go too far – there had to be some benefit to him and any more government attempts to restrict his access to certain benefits would be pushing it too far. He saw it as a bargain in which there had to be some returns. At the time of the interview there had been speculation about so called 'affluence testing' of certain benefits with child benefit being one of them. Of this, he said:

If you're not careful you're taxing the earners highly to provide the benefits for the unemployed. So it's a matter of getting a balance, I think, so it's a reasonable deal for everyone? I don't think I'd be too happy at losing the child benefit and then being taxed at 50% for instance, I'd feel that was a bad deal for me personally. Or if tax relief on pensions was withdrawn, I think the current government are probably restricting some of the benefits for me, in some of those areas.

Another AB respondent said: 'You just wonder what do you pay your taxes for. I mean National Insurance for, because there's less and less that you're getting back, there's less and less payback.' Changes to help to home owners with mortgage payments in the event of unemployment also concerned a number of respondents who felt that the change in the rules was designed to encourage them to take out private provision. One C home owner said:

We've got things like stakeholder pensions coming in, mortgage protection policies, personal pensions, that sort of thing. And things like restrictions on mortgage interest payments for home owners under income support – I mean, I think that was a very tough measure, but it was purely designed to save money by making people take out their own provision.

There was a common feeling that 'welfare' was changing and that more self provision was inevitable. This person echoed what another AB respondent had to say about 'welfare' more broadly. They were happy to pay more tax if it was going to be spent on education and health but they were not happy with increases in social security spending. He thought that restricting his access to social security by for example affluence testing child benefit would mean that 'the middle classes who work bloody hard will be penalized and those who haven't worked will be laughing.' In contrast, a very small minority in each socio-economic group thought that benefit levels were too low and were happy to see them increase and if need be pay higher taxes. There was a recognition that the state would always be needed to provide a basic safety net. An AB technician said:

> I'm quite happy paying my national insurance contributions knowing that somebody is getting some use out of them. I've no grievances with that at all. It's dead easy for somebody who is competent at providing for themselves but there's a lot of people that aren't, a lot of people haven't got the same get up and go, they need benefits, they need national health insurance, they need it.

Policy implications: undermining support for social security?

With a few exceptions, the ways in which people talked about social security were highly individualistic and negative. In spite of this, there was almost universal support for the idea that the state should provide at least some help to the unemployed. However, it would be a mistake to assume that the negativity about social security and claimants meant that people were positive about private alternatives. Those who could afford to and had made private provision had done so because they felt that social security would not be an effective backstop for them and that there was a certain inevitability about the need to make more private provision rather than relying on the state. Amongst Cs and Ds most, though not all, thought that the state should provide for those who were unemployed.

Despite this, social security benefits were not seen or discussed in positive terms. The dual challenges to social security of its very negative image and the questioning of whether it represents a good bargain for the better off, pose real threats to those for whom private alternatives are not available. Walker (1998) has turned the arguments about social security around and argued that spending in this area has been the support mechanism for the deregulation of the economy and the flexibilization of the labour market. He makes a very different case for recognition of social security as a common good:

> Social security needs to be recognised for what it is; evidence of a civilised and civilising society; a reward for past contributions and an investment in people and society's future prosperity. Since the vast majority of benefit recipients are neither malingerers nor guilty of fraud or abuse, benefits should be designed, promoted and delivered primarily to foster the well-being of the many, rather than to frustrate the despicable activities of the few.
>
> (Walker 1998)

However, there is currently very little 'talking up' of social security as a social good in the way that Walker describes. Lister (this volume) recounts Tony Blair's remarks in a Beveridge lecture in which he described how the welfare state had become associated with 'fraud, abuse, laziness, a dependency culture, social irresponsibility encouraged by welfare dependency'. She argues that his Government's own approach to social security has done little to redress the negative ways in which both the system and benefit claimants are perceived. In the July 2000 Government spending review, one of the main boasts was that higher spending on public services had been made possible in large part by the dramatic reduction in money which had to be spent on debt and on social security. This study suggests that although state support for the unemployed remains largely intact, the respondents in this study were not on the whole persuaded that more money needed to be spent on social security. There was a tacit acceptance that the state simply would not in the future meet the obligations towards the unemployed that it once had. This is unsurprising given the way that the model of the future welfare state is often discussed. David Blunkett in a recent speech to the Institute for Public Policy Research argued that families might have to take more responsibility for themselves in the event of unemployment:

> But it is not possible for us to create an environment in which the state has some overarching responsibility for paying people who are not at work. We must ensure the balance between the responsibility of the family and that of the state is recognised, and that we do not fall into the trap of believing that we can overcome the structural inequalities of all families in all communities.

The unwillingness to engage with structural obstacles to successful strategies to deal with an event like unemployment means that once again many families living on the edges of work and benefits are in a precarious and potentially excluded position. The evidence clearly shows a considerable number of families in D, as well as C, social classes who, while they were only too aware of increasing risks, were not in a position to protect themselves from such risks due simply to a lack of money. Even where some households had some scope for planning, a hierarchy of risk meant that planning against the risk of unemployment was not possible when higher priorities such as life insurances and pensions had been met. An examination of the financial planning of all socio-economic groups reveals a clear pattern of prioritizing certain risks over others. Many respondents, both those who had the ability to plan, as well as those who were expressing a desire to plan, placed planning for death at the top of the list when they had children. After this came planning for retirement. A significant minority had planned or wanted to plan for the eventuality of illness or accident to protect their income. The risk of unemployment came below all the other risks as a priority. This appeared to be because people viewed the impact of the other risks as potentially much more damaging than unemployment. This is not to say that many people did not fear unemployment, or given unlimited funds, would not have planned for this; rather that it was not a first priority. They also felt better prepared to face unemployment than other life events, either through savings or protection within their employment, through their skills and employability, or because the market would always require workers for poor jobs.

Policy-makers need to consider very carefully the lack of available income in some households to plan for the future and the very real priorities that people have which are reflected in their decisions about what it is most important for them to plan for. Those that had some money to spare needed products which were flexible and took into account that there were times when they had a little extra money and times when they did not. At present, low income households have little choice but to be reliant on state support at times of unemployment, yet present policy refuses to acknowledge this, continuing to cut back on state protection, particularly for unemployed home owners, leaving many effectively unprotected by either the state or private safety nets.

At the time of writing, a high street bank was running a poster campaign asking 'who'll put food on the table if I lose my job?', and offering a range of income protection products. It is unsurprising that people feel that they will have to make more provision. Yet it is entirely unclear on what these assumptions are based and it leaves those whose only real choice in the face of limited resources is social security, at risk of becoming even more marginalized from the rest of society. In the absence of a challenge to the image of social security as a social ill, it seems as if private provision becomes almost by default the natural and attractive option although there is no evidence that it is presently, or will in the future prove, effective or reliable for those who can afford to take it (Taylor-Gooby *et al*. 1999). Private, market solutions to social policy problems like unemployment are largely untried. They work least well for those most at risk and least able to protect themselves. A growing body of work is evaluating the effectiveness of policies like MPPI and finding serious gaps in the protections they afford (e.g. Kempson *et al*. 1999). Furthermore, the empirical evidence supports a growing body of work which demonstrates that, even if the necessary resources are available, people are not as keen to seek out individualized solutions as the Government and many other commentators might suppose. Many retain a belief in the efficacy of state provision and a scepticism about the ability of the private sector to protect them (Burchardt *et al*. 1999; Ford, 1999; Taylor-Gooby *et al*. 1999; Williams *et al*. 1999).

The evidence in this study is that those who increasingly see social security as a bad deal for them are actively asking questions about opting out. Private provision has clearly been ear marked by commerce and government as the way ahead for some. A recent Unicef (2000) report argues that focusing on the market to alleviate poverty will not prove effective overall and is critical of the British Government's reliance on paid work. The report called for the adequacy of benefits to be re-examined, but our respondents' sentiments about social security and the approach of Government make that task look a formidable one. Whilst the Government's renewed emphasis on work has to be welcomed, evidence suggests that it is not enough. Is the Government also willing to afford security to those who work in low paid, stressful jobs, with very few occupational advantages enjoyed by other socio-economic groups, thereby offering families a more secure base from which they could realistically plan for the future? In the meantime, current policy leaves a large proportion of individuals, particularly those in the lower socio-economic groups, vulnerable to the impacts of a flexible labour market whilst the better off purchase their safety and freedom from risk.

Note

1   The authors would like to acknowledge the Economic and Social Research Council for funding this work as part of their Risk and Human Behaviour Programme (Award Reference Number L211 25 2054). The research team also included Janet Ford (Centre for Housing Policy, University of York), and Andreas Cebulla, Sue Middleton, Simon Roberts and Robert Walker (Centre for Research in Social Policy, Loughborough University).

References

Blunkett, D. (2000) 'On Your Side': The New Welfare State as the Engine of Economic Prosperity. Speech to the Institute of Public Policy Research, 7 June at http://www.dfee.gov.uk/Dbspeech070600/index.htm and reported in A. Grice (2000) 'Blunkett hints at end to unemployment benefit', The Independent, 8 June.

Burchardt, T., Hills, J. and Propper, C. (1999) Private Welfare and Public Policy, York: York Publishing Services.

Cebulla, A., Abbott, D., Ford, J., Middleton, S., Quilgars, D. and Walker, R. (1998) 'A Geography of Insurance Exclusion – Perceptions of Unemployment Risk and Actuarial Risk Assessment'. Paper presented to the Second European Urban and Regional Studies Conference, University of Durham, September 1998.

Cebulla, A. and Ford, J. (2000) 'Confronting Unemployment: Families' Management of Risk in the Flexible Labour Market'. Economic and Social Research Council Risk and Human Behaviour Newsletter. Summer.

Department of Environment, Transport and Regions (2000) Quality and Choice: A Decent Home for All: The Housing Green Paper, London: DETR.

Department of Social Security (1998) A New Contract for Welfare, London: HMSO.

Department of Trade and Industry (1998) Fairness at Work, Cm 3968. London: HMSO.

Esping-Anderson, G. (1996) Welfare States in Transition: National Adaptations in Global Economics, London: Sage.

Ford, J. (1999) 'Risk and the Failure of Social Capital: Home Owners and Private Mortgage Insurance'. Paper presented to the Social Policy Association Annual Conference, July 1999.

HM Treasury (1997) The Modernisation of Britain's Tax and Benefit System: Employment Opportunity in a Changing Labour Market, London: HMSO.

Kempson, E., Ford, J., Quilgars, D. and Whylie, C. (1999) Unsafe Safety Nets, York: Centre for Housing Policy, University of York.

Lindley, R. and Wilson, R. (1998) Review of the Economy and Employment, 1997/8, Coventry: Institute of Employment Research, University of Warwick.

Quilgars, D. and Abbott, D. (2000) 'Working in the risk society: families perceptions of, and response to, flexible labour markets and the restructuring of welfare', *Community, Work and Family* 3(1): 15–36.

Taylor-Gooby, P., Dean, H., Munro, M. and Parker, G. (1999). 'Risk and the Welfare State', *British Journal of Sociology* 50(2): 177–95.

Unicef (2000) *A League Table of Child Poverty in Rich Nations*. http://www.unicef-icdc.org/pdf/poverty.pdf

Walker, R. (1998) 'Promoting positive welfare', *New Economy* 5(2): 77–82.

Williams, T., Hill, M. and Davies, R. (1999) *Attitudes to the Welfare State and the Response to Reform*, Leeds: Department of Social Security.

Chapter 9

Managing the body

Competing approaches to risk assessment in community care

Kathryn Ellis and Ann Davis

This chapter brings together theoretical and empirical work on differing modes of risk assessment deployed within community care by policy-makers, professionals and service users. Drawing upon work developed elsewhere (Ellis 1999a), the first section outlines three successive welfare regimes, constituted around the corporeal discourses of 'physical efficiency', 'social efficiency' and the 'independent body', and the modes of risk assessment with which they are associated. Community care emerged after the Second World War as a means of sharing social risks and the second section describes its origins and subsequent transformation into a mechanism for protecting the state from dependency – or preventing dependency from ever arising (Ellis 1999b). Yet discourses are neither unified in their content nor uniform in their effects but offer oppositional spaces for strategic action (Turner 1996: 173). In the final section, we draw on the findings of a study of needs assessment within the new community care (Davis *et al*. 1997) to reveal competing definitions of and strategies for assessing risk amongst the actors involved.

Risk assessment and bodily welfare regimes

The concept of corporeal welfare regimes draws on a wider tradition of viewing the body as the medium through which social order and institutions are maintained. As Schatzki and Natter point out, a common theme uniting the work of theorists such as Pierre Bourdieu, Mary Douglas, Michel Foucault and John O'Neill is 'the dependency of the perpetuation of bodies sociopolitical on the production of socioculturated bodies cut to certain specifications'. Nor, they argue, is it just bodies which are tailored, but 'individuals (subjects) – human beings with particular identities, genders, characters, joys, understandings and the like' (1996: 2–3). This section outlines the way in which particular welfare subjects have been constructed under the three regimes as a means of managing risks to the dominant social and economic order.

Physical efficiency

The involvement of welfare systems in producing 'socioculturated bodies' can be analysed in terms of Foucault's 'bio-power', or 'power over bodies and by bodies' (Hewitt 1991: 230). Bio-power is created both through the discipline of the individual body – or 'anatomo-politics' – and through 'bio-politics' – or the regulation of whole populations (Foucault 1979). Anatomo-politics can be traced to the incorporation of the clinical gaze into a range of scientific disciplines that served to classify and normalize human behaviour within the increasingly urban spaces of early industrial capitalism. Disciplinary power spread through the prison and various prison-like establishments, including the workhouse and specialist medical institutions set up under the 1834 Poor Law (Amendment) Act, to render politically dangerous bodies 'docile', productive and economically useful. By the second phase of industrial capitalism from the 1880s onwards, statistical science had shifted the disciplinary gaze from abnormal groups to the normality of the population as a whole. Welfare interventions were driven by the norms of 'physical efficiency' in line with bio-political concerns to secure the health, welfare and productivity of the mass of labouring bodies.

In the latter part of the nineteenth century, the bio-politics of public health enabled risks to physical efficiency to be predicted, or managed over time as well as in space. Armstrong (1993) points out that, once it became known that risks to health could no longer be hygienically contained within external places, the 'quarantine model' of public health was displaced by 'sanitary science'. The knowledge that health hazards could penetrate the boundaries of the body pre-cipitated a range of measures to sanitize the space between the physical body and external environment. By the early twentieth century, when the principles of germ theory had established that health risks were directly spread between people, a new form of risk assessment emerged in the 'Dispensary gaze' which brought whole populations under the surveillance of the tuberculosis dispensary, the venereal disease clinic, the school medical service inspection clinic, the child welfare clinic (Armstrong 1983). Not only were the origins of illness relocated in the community rather than in the body of the individual, but the physical space between bodies was transformed into a social space governable through welfare action.

The extent to which threats to physical efficiency came to be seen both as located within the social rather than the physical body, and as increasingly preventable, is illustrated by other forms of welfare emerging in this period. A limited form of welfare citizenship was introduced to avert the danger of socialism (Thane 1982). Threats to the physical fitness on which military strength and heavy industrial production depended were confronted by eugenicist measures to prevent the reproduction of those deviating from the desired physical and moral average (Davis 1995). Working-class mothers were denied full social rights but invested with new skills and powers to enhance the physical efficiency of the future workforce (Williams 1989), even as the policing of unhygienic behaviours in the home and family brought their domestic lives under increasing supervision (Donzelot 1979).

Social efficiency

Giddens (1994) identifies the politics of 'risk-sharing' as the inspiration behind the formation of the welfare state, arguing that notions of risk as opposed to fate imply an ethics as they suggest that economic and social life not only can but also should be humanely controlled. According to Armstrong (1983), the integrated community within which the new bio-politics flourished was the creation of the medico-social survey, a mode of mass regulation which emerged during the Second World War to satisfy the need to know and make visible bodily hazards in a community under threat. After the war, Keynesian demand management was directed at overcoming the hazards of an unstable market economy in order to sustain consumption and full employment, while a system of social security protected citizens against 'states of dependency' (Titmuss 1963).

Thus the burgeoning apparatus of welfare was directed at ensuring the efficiency of the social body itself, rather than simply the physical efficiency of bodies within social spaces. Social efficiency was secured by redistributing the normal social risks encountered by thrifty, hard-working citizens according to the principle of universality but only selectively assisting the 'abnormal', such as those outside the labour market. Reshaping the interior spaces of the body of welfare subjects served both to reinforce normalcy and contain the costs of social reproduction. Thus an ethos of productivism privileged industry as the bearer of moral meaning and harnessed the male breadwinner to the imperatives of mass production (Giddens 1994), while an ideology of familism, combined with moral panics about the hazards of 'maternal deprivation', positioned married women as housewives and mothers rather than as paid workers.

Independent body

From the mid-1970s onwards, the restructuring of paid work and family life disrupted traditional certainties even as the emergence of a plurality of contested knowledges eroded active forms of trust (Giddens 1991). Beck (1992) argued that the definition and management of risk had become so pervasive under advanced capitalism as to create 'risk societies' particularly, as Giddens (1994) points out, once the ecological hazards of global capitalism had added 'manufactured' risk to the 'external' risks of birth, sickness, old age and death.

Giddens (1994) argued that disruptions to the predictability of the lifecourse made it less feasible for welfare states to offer social protection against the external risks of birth, sickness, old age and death or to provide 'precautionary aftercare' for dependent groups. As Petersen points out, both Giddens and Beck view people living in post-traditional societies as autonomous actors who shape their own biography on the basis of pragmatic calculations of risk and opportunity (1997: 92). At the centre of this increased reflexivity is the consumption ethic which encourages people to negotiate lifestyles in line with the possibilities of the marketplace. In Britain, the neo-liberal project of the incoming Conservative government in 1979 articulated with growing social reflexivity, and the attendant individualization of risk and opportunity. Welfare systems were reconstituted by the corporeal discourse of the 'independent body', individualizing and recommodifying formerly collectivized risks in line with the dictates of competitiveness and profitability.

Yet welfare restructuring reflected the contradictory demands of post-industrial capitalism. Economic competitiveness requires, on the one hand, the promotion of consumption and the stimulation of desire and, on the other, the higher productivity of a disciplined workforce and ascetic restraint. Early strategies of privatization and low direct taxation, pursued by Conservative administrations in the 1980s, articulated with the consumption ethic, and the subsequent marketization of welfare systems promised greater consumer choice. Yet fiscal probity also demanded that quasi-markets were efficient and delivered value for money which required the regulatory hand of the manager to temper the play of competitive forces.

Contradictory demands were also made on the welfare subject. Entrepreneurial individuals were urged to secure their risk-free futures by using market freedoms to take risks in the here and now (Rose 1993). Yet the privileged social identity was that of the self-caring citizen-consumer who avoided dependency through hard work and prudent protection against lifecourse contingencies. Moreover, to the extent that men occupy a privileged position in the paid economy, as Culpitt points out: 'This depiction of risk as a marketplace "reality" is, quintessentially, a masculine view of the world' (1999: 78).

Health provides a powerful metaphor for the cultural contradictions of late capitalism (Crawford 1984). Consumption has both transformed the body into the principal vehicle of desire and fostered the notion that its exchange value can be enhanced by reshaping it in line with idealized images of youth, fitness and beauty (Falk 1994; Giddens 1992; Shilling 1993). Sickness, impairment and ageing threaten the body beautiful whose exterior and interior must be protected by 'bodily maintenance' regimes (Featherstone 1991). To the extent that health is dependent on intentional acts, such as diet and exercise, the healthy body has come to signify worthiness as a person, evidencing foresight, self-control, hard work and personal responsibility, whilst moral deviants, who voluntarily abuse their bodies, represent a new form of depravity (Lupton 1994).

In neo-liberal welfare states, preoccupations with the surface appearance of the body, and its attendant concerns with bodily maintenance, have been harnessed by the bio-politics of health promotion. Carter describes preventative medicine as a form of risk assessment based on probabilistic reasoning which, by identifying the risk factors associated with future illness, transforms an uncertain future into one which individuals can control by making rational choices about their lifestyle. Preventative health regimes offer a means not simply of containing the cost of future dependency, but also of controlling transgressions between safe and dangerous places by identifying and governing the dangerous 'other' in the interests of the 'same' (Carter 1995: 140–5).

Community care, risk and the body

Social efficiency and the emergence of community care

Coming into general use in the 1950s and early 1960s, the term 'community care' reflects the ambiguous conceptualization of the body within medico-welfare discourses of 'social efficiency' and associated modes of risk assessment. On the one hand, the social space surrounding bodies – the 'community' – constituted normalcy. Thus, in dismantling the institutional apparatus of the Poor Law, the 1948 National Assistance Act (NAA) confirmed the local community as the rightful place for older and disabled people. The depersonalizing effects of institutional life were challenged in new discourses around labelling, stigma and 'institutionalization', while a discourse of normalization identified the formerly abnormal as 'really normal'. The politics of risk sharing supported civil rights campaigns on behalf of people 'wrongly' confined to mental hospitals and the subsequent struggles of people with physical impairments against their segregation.

On the other hand, the risks of dependency were controlled by identifying bodies requiring 'care and attention' under the 1948 NAA according to a normal/abnormal dichotomy. In the case of older people, degrees of bodily dependency formed the basis for determining the point at which local authority beds should substitute for costly hospital beds (Means 1995). This principle of 'substitutability', as Levick (1992) points out, was routinely deployed as a means of holding the costs of community care in check. Thus legal powers to provide a full range of domiciliary services to older people were initially withheld for fear they would be improperly substituted for family care (Means 1995). Disabled people's dependency was increasingly managed by substituting the needs claims of individual bodies for rights claims on the social body. The 1970 Chronically Sick and Disabled Persons Act simultaneously upheld people's rights to occupy ordinary social spaces, whilst endorsing the provision of 'special' services in, yet segregated from, the community. Eligibility for services was linked via the anatomo-politics of needs assessment to tests of physical and mental functioning.

Within the 'bureau-professional regimes' of the post-war welfare state (Newman and Clarke 1994), however, community care was not only distributed rationally, according to administrative techniques of 'objective necessity' (Hill and Bramley 1986: 58), but flexibly according to professional needs assessments. Professional training in psychological theories and therapeutic methodology opened up psychic and social spaces between people, equipping social workers to build relationships and uncover the needs of the unique individual (Aldridge 1996; Dominelli 1996). The Seebohm Report (Cmnd 3703) on the 'personal social services' represents the high-water mark of both social efficiency and social work. Bolstered by generic social work, the social services department offered a 'single door' through which the local community could access a unified service, whilst social workers promoted social cohesion by bringing about adaptive change in individuals, in their social relationships and in the social environment (Webb and Wistow 1987).

In the event, confusion over the principle and practice of genericism (Bamford 1990) perpetuated specialisms which, in the case of disabled people, were organized around the anatomical body. Older people, typically perceived as less capable of change and development, were frequently excluded from the psycho-social gaze of the professional social worker with interventions characterized by surveillance rather than direct work (Hughes and Mtezuka 1992: 233). More generally, it was administrative rather than professional categorizations of need which dominated the post-Seebohm departments (Blaxter 1976; Smith 1980).

The 'independent body' and the restructuring of community care

In the 1970s, as fiscal crisis enmeshed with panics about the 'demographic time-bomb' of an ageing population, bio-politics were dominated by the task of managing the 'burden of care'. The community was redefined within neo-liberal orthodoxy as the source of care rather than the social and geographical spaces within which caring took place. Over the 1980s the highly cost-effective strategy of 'supporting the carer' took shape as the 'informal carer' gained prominence in policy documents (Twigg and Atkin 1994). Upholding the rights of disabled people, newly outlined in the 1986 Disabled Persons (Services, Representation and Consultation) Act, was an altogether riskier proposition for local authorities facing charge- and expenditure-capping. The Conservative government argued that, in any case, the unimplemented sections were superseded by its planned reforms of community care, promising as they did a new kind of right: consumer sovereignty.

In practice, the new mixed economy of care ushered in by the 1990 National Health Service and Community Care Act (NHSCCA) reflected characteristically contradictory objectives. As Langan and Clarke point out, competition introduced by the market-based logic of the purchaser–provider split was designed both to enhance the quality and choice of care and to offer better value for money by exposing and reducing costs (1994: 78). Local authority managers had to transform bureau-professional regimes into 'enterprise' cultures (Aldridge 1996), whilst simultaneously obeying the logic of McDonaldization in contracting arrangements. Inasmuch as the production of highly specific products by a plurality of organizations depended on standardizing patterns of production and consumption, Hadley and Clough (1996) claim that the factory or industrial model of care came to dominate the quasi-markets of community care.

Consumption was routinized through assessment and care management systems, set up to tackle the new demands of risk assessment, that is to protect the state from dependency – or prevent states of dependency from ever arising. Pilot care management systems developed by the Personal Social Services Research Unit at the University of Kent suggested the need for a degree of 'downward substitution' at the interface between institutional and home-based care if people were to be maintained in the least dependent setting (Challis 1992). Local authorities were required to prioritize the needs of the most dependent who were also at risk of entering institutional care because of the lack of – or apparent fragility of – informal support. Despite the rhetoric of needs-based assessments, they were effectively instructed to define need in terms of service criteria which should 'allow through just enough people with needs exactly to use up their budget (or be prepared to adjust their budgets)' (Audit Commission 1993, para. 15). The Seebohm principle of universality was replaced by the pragmatics of explicit targeting.

Assessing capacity for self-care, both in terms of ability to pay and bodily functioning, was central to the management of dependency. With the implementation of charging policies based on the 'economic cost' of services, a turnstile was erected at the single door. Independence was seen less in terms of pursuing valued personal goals through long-term work, than in terms of bodily competence. Given the expectation that services would intervene no more than necessary to promote independence (Department of Health 1989, para. 1.8–1.10), bodily independence was positioned both as an aspect of eligibility and a service objective. Risk/need matrices scrutinized the vulnerable body for signs of ill health, inability to perform the tasks of daily living unaided, poor mobility and so on to establish which bodily needs should be satisfied, and for how long, if independent functioning was to be maintained or restored.

Care for those who failed to avoid dependency was minimized by limiting service provision to 'life and limb' protection for the already vulnerable. Whereas the medico-social gaze sought out those at risk in the community by maintaining surveillance over the still healthy, the preventative role of domiciliary services was eclipsed by an increasingly narrow focus on personal care and by the return of housework, shopping and 'pop-in' services to the private sector. Recommodifying the social spaces around and between bodies revealed a multiplicity of independent bodies, justifying the relegation of 'social' need to the lower echelons of need hierarchies. Holidays and other social activities were abandoned whilst access to services designed to prevent the risk of social isolation were increasingly restricted by charging (Sainsbury 1995: 192–3).

Minimizing dependency also called for the production of care to be routinized in ways which have displaced forms of welfare based on the quality of human relationships (Hadley and Clough 1996). Household arrangements were regularized by the managerial gaze to prevent unauthorized 'dependencies', that is, the informal arrangements that used to build up over time between home help and client. The construction of 'users' and 'carers' as separate cost and assessment units denies the reciprocity of caring relationships, reinforced by 'packages of care' which specify the carer's labour in tending the dependent body in the stead of or on behalf of the state. Caring is stripped of its inter-subjectivity as those tasks which cannot be counted or costed are rendered invisible (Brown and Smith 1993: 188), and the body is transformed into an object to be cared for rather than a subject to be cared about.

The psychosocial techniques of social work similarly required reworking in line with new modes of risk assessment. The purchaser–provider split fractured the holism of the professional assessment, comprising both initial stage of 'diagnosis' and subsequent design of appropriate interventions. Official guidance on assessment and care management further denied a distinct role for social work by the determined reference to an all-embracing 'practitioner' (Cheetham 1993: 157). Professional status relates to 'person-focused' rather than 'resource-based' objectives (Hugman 1994: 245), yet new arrangements were designed less as a process of human interaction than as a linear sequence of interrelated decisions about eligibility. New technology underlined the transformation of the professional assessment into an 'administrative' task (Hughes 1995: 142), providing 'invisible monitoring systems' which laid practitioners' actions open to managerial scrutiny and ensured their compliance with service criteria and budgetary disciplines (Newman and Clarke 1994: 20).

In the next section we draw on the findings of an empirical investigation into the negotiation of access to a community care needs assessment to explore competing approaches to risk assessment amongst practitioners and service users.

Community care in practice: competing approaches to risk assessment

The research was conducted in 1995–96, two years after full implementation of the 1990 NHSCCA. Detailed guidance from the Audit Commission and Social Services Inspectorate (SSI) underlined a determinedly top-down approach towards implementing new assessment and care management systems and formed a highly rationalistic blueprint against which local action could be measured (Lewis and Glennerster 1996: 18). Yet previous research (Ellis 1993) suggested that, however rational the official account, the informal practices of front-line practitioners would be significant at point of entry to new systems. Our study was therefore based on observations of assessment practice in six social work teams in two local authority social services departments. In addition, interviews were conducted with fifty disabled people and twenty-three carers who had had some assessment contact with these teams (see Davis *et al.* 1997 for full account).

The front-line practitioners

According to operational manuals inspected as part of our study, a common set of procedures and eligibility criteria had been adopted across each authority, based on dominant modes of risk assessment. Yet, as SSI guidelines warned, 'Agencies and professions tend to vary in their perceptions of risk and crisis' (1991: 59). We found that, in practice, three distinct approaches to risk assessment were adopted depending on the position of the social work team within assessment and care management systems and associated levels of demand. As 'gatekeepers', the two community-based *generic* teams and the *hospital* team screened high levels of referrals and also operated within tight budgets. In contrast, the three *specialist* teams for people with physical and sensory impairments were not only protected from high bombardment rates but enjoyed access to resources outside the limited menu of services supplied or funded by the local authority.

The generic teams relied most heavily on departmental risk/need matrices when assessing the relative priority of referrals. Decisions were typically made on the basis of the paperwork, supplemented by follow-up 'phone calls to other professionals, prospective users and relatives. Professional discourses were occasionally deployed as social workers voiced their suspicions that 'grief', 'loss' or 'family conflicts' lurked beneath the referral information, yet concerns were only followed up if available evidence could also be matched to prioritization criteria. Inasmuch as 'initial assessments' could be added to the tally of completed assessments, practitioners had little incentive to engage in face-to-face work. Indeed it was not unusual for fairly detailed assessments to be conducted over the 'phone without the knowledge of the person being 'assessed'.

As Castel (1991) observes, managing danger in contemporary neo-liberal societies is less about confining dangerous individuals, or controlling them in face-to-face relationships with experts, than about profiling risk to prevent its occurrence. Social workers on the generic teams mobilized assessment technology defensively to avoid the danger of wasting valuable time uncovering needs at variance with risk-based criteria or the limited menu of services to which they gave access. The completion of computer screens demarcating each stage of assessment and care management *during* the initial stages of assessment, rather than off-line as on other teams, tied their invisible calculations of risk even more securely to departmental criteria.

On the hospital team, persistent injunctions to avoid 'bed-blocking' meant that date of discharge played a prominent part in the prioritization of referrals. Yet the particularly vulnerable body of the patient required safe as well as speedy dispatch. In detailed enquiries made prior to a ward visit, social workers relied heavily on clinical assessments of bodily hazards, generally forming a judgement about risk, and therefore eligibility, before they reached the bedside. During assessment visits, if patients articulated needs which fell outside the team's stock response, they tended to go unacknowledged or were converted into a need for services provided or funded by the authority, particularly home care.

Despite the apparently narrow scope of its work, the hospital team saw the safe discharge of patients, often at short notice, as a means of practising effectively and responsively as social workers. Their sense of professional identity was reinforced by the pride they took in protecting the rights of social services clients within the hospital setting. Their advocacy was required to prevent hospital staff from compromising patients' autonomy by overestimating the level of intervention required on discharge, or, conversely, from exerting undue pressure to effect a discharge before the appropriate clinical and social assessments were carried out or against relatives' wishes.

The specialist teams had more time and other resources at their disposal than the other teams, as well as a greater awareness of, and commitment to, disability rights. Widely ignored elsewhere, disabled people's entitlement to a comprehensive assessment, extant under previous legislation, was recognized by these teams. Risk-based eligibility criteria were used to decide the order in which, rather than whether, people would be assessed. In contrast to the defensive tactics deployed elsewhere – underlining the scarcity of resources, suggesting people sought help privately, using charging policies as an informal tool of rationing, attempting to redefine needs in terms of available services – social workers on the specialist teams felt freer to enter into open-ended discussions about need, underlined by a philosophy of providing sufficient information to enable people to take an active part in assessment. Where gaps in provision were identified, which undermined people's ability to live ordinary lives in the community, these were recorded as unmet need.

The assessment strategies adopted by the generic and hospital teams, who located risk both in the vulnerable body and in levels of bombardment, were effectively based on the identification of 'safe options' (Lawson 1996: 52). Despite expressed concerns about deprofessionalization, in practice, social workers acted as 'street-level bureaucrats', using tactics which enabled them to manage demand and maintain an even flow of work (see Ellis *et al.* 1999). Given that risk and risk-taking were viewed as part of everyday living and, indeed, as essential to personal growth and self-determination, social workers on the specialist teams were more willing to respond to the risk assessments and strategies of risk management adopted by disabled people and carers.

The users

So far as the people we interviewed were concerned, or whose assessments we observed, danger formed part of the daily fabric of their lives. Fears about failing health, relationship breakdown, entry into residential care or death were often heightened by social isolation and the anxiety of managing on limited incomes in poor accommodation and in neighbourhoods where crime was perceived as a constant threat. Yet these concerns were likely to be discounted or deflected during contacts with social work teams as they could not be readily accommodated within the narrow formulations of risk on which eligibility criteria and assessment check-lists were based.

Even securing help to manage risky situations was a bit of a lottery. Information about services had often been obtained by accident – a chance remark by a friend or neighbour, a voluntary organization leaflet pushed through the door, a conversation across a hospital ward, the meals-on-wheels delivered to a neighbour. Functional fragmentation made it difficult for enquirers to find their way into community care systems and there appeared to be little co-ordination between different teams and sections. Moreover each time a fresh enquiry was made the route seemed to change. Once contact was made, the response was hardly welcoming. An interviewee summed up several recent attempts thus: 'As you start talking to social services they're immediately thinking of an excuse and where to send you.'

The economic rationality underlying risk assessment systems not only appeared highly irrational to interviewees but threw up new hazards, such as the cost to people in poor health and on low incomes of conducting assessments over the telephone. Charging policies posed an additional threat. People often refused to accept an assessment for fear of incurring future charges, whilst the cost of existing services meant that, far from increasing people's sense of security, it had left some fearful of any future escalation in their needs. The fear of losing the family home to pay for residential care was another commonly perceived threat associated with contacting social services departments.

According to Giddens (1991), risk assessment is a means of 'colonising the future' in an uncertain world. Similarly, many of the people we interviewed had expected their community care assessment to secure a bridgehead into the particularly hazardous territory of their futures. Contact with a specialist team did frequently provide useful strategies for managing present and future situations, as well as opening up a reassuring channel of communication for future use. For long-term users, contact with a known and trusted professional provided a valued sense of security. Contacts with other teams, however, were more frequently ephemeral, confusing and often alienating. An interviewee identified the unspoken question underlying her recent social work assessment as: 'What are you trying to get out of social services?', especially as it had been emphasized that she would have to pay for any services.

People who thought they were 'too able-bodied', or who sought other types of support, had been deterred from seeking further help by the knowledge that the new community care centred on personal care for the highly dependent. However, many people did share practitioners' concern to minimize the risks associated with bodily vulnerability. The hazards of bathing safely, whilst safeguarding privacy, were frequently raised during interviews, as were strategies such as staying in the familiar environment of the home to avoid falls or preparing only simple meals using convenience foods to avoid scalds and burns. Yet, because the basis of their risk analysis differed from that of service managers, people sometimes concluded that the costs of accepting services outweighed any potential benefits.

Carter argues that dominant modes of risk assessment represent an attempt to settle on a preferred outcome by comparing alternative courses of action 'across the dimensions of probability and value' (1995: 137). In terms of value, access to community care is governed by calculations of the risk of non-intervention at given levels of dependency. Yet if people felt that any increase in security was outweighed by the risk of losing valued independence, they would refuse services in order to protect the integrity of the body and domestic space. In terms of probabilistic reasoning, purchasers routinized patterns of production and consumption in order to anticipate the costs of care. Yet people managing fluctuating illnesses were necessarily present-oriented and therefore unable to predict the type and level of support they might require at any given time, or else fearful of tying themselves down to onerous routines.

Even if services were accepted, these had not always minimized risk. Long delays in supplying aids and adaptations perpetuated the hazards people faced in using stairs or bathing, or in lifting relatives. Home care staff could not always be relied upon to turn up at the specified times. Hospital discharge was a particularly worrying time, and several people complained of returning home without the expected provision in place. Sometimes services exposed users to new hazards. Constant changes of staff, drawn from a range of private and statutory agencies, not only necessitated wearisome repetitions of caring routines but also heightened people's fear of the dangerous stranger.

Conclusion

As part of a wider restructuring of the welfare state in the 1980s, shifts in community care were designed to counter threats to economic rather than social efficiency. The body was reconstituted as a 'burden' and as an object to be cared for in isolation rather than as a subject to be cared about through preventative and continuous care in the community. Powered by risk-based prioritization criteria, rationalized systems of assessment and care management were geared towards minimizing the costs of dependency. Practitioners were enabled both to scrutinize the intimate bodily functions and needs of 'users' and to interrogate their 'carers' as the basis for allocating time-limited packages of care and disciplining carers into taking on their share of the burden of care.

Risk/need matrices represent risk as the negative consequences of not intervening to prevent harm to vulnerable bodies, mirroring the predominantly negative treatment of risk in contemporary risk society as the probability of adversity (Douglas 1990). This is a defensive stance commonly shared by welfare professionals, particularly where older people are concerned (Reed 1998). Yet Alaszewski maintains that the possibility for more open practice exists if professionals are empowered to act as 'risk managers', collaborating with service users in balancing the positive and negative outcomes of risk (1998: 147). In our own study, only the specialist teams approximated this approach. Working with service users' own cost–benefit risk analyses, social workers tried to ensure that people were both protected from harmful risks and enabled to take positive risks.

In the face of over-protectiveness on the part of clinical staff, social workers on the hospital team were keenly aware of the need to balance patients' autonomy against their particular vulnerability to harmful risks, yet powerless in the face of limited time and other resources to respond to people's own risk assessments. Risk assessments conducted by the generic teams, who dealt predominantly with the largest client group of older people, were driven by departmental prioritization criteria. As Reed points out, the risk-taking behaviour of older people is frequently based on trade-offs between living 'unsafe' but better quality lives (1998: 248–9). Ironically, in the new mixed economy of care, not only do protective services create new risks, but risk-based criteria screen out precisely those preventative services which would enable people to strike the desired balance between safety and autonomy. Practitioners on the generic teams also managed the additional risk of intervening unnecessarily, and the attendant costs of dependency, in a particularly powerful form. Their rationing strategies cut across people's own risk analyses, whilst leaving them further exposed to hazardous situations.

Whilst the corporeal discourses of welfare powerfully shape people's experience of community care, the circulation of competing discourses of risk amongst policy-makers, front-line professionals and service users reveals that they are also open to challenge and change. As Williams and Bendelow explain: 'Discourses . . . are embodied, and social institutions cannot be understood apart from the real, lived experiences and actions of bodies' (1998: 65). Social reflexivity has led to the articulation of new corporealities and embodied subjectivities by feminists, the disability movement, gay activists. Disability activists, who have relocated 'disability' in social barriers rather than bodily impairment, draw upon discourses of inclusive citizenship and interdependence to argue for rights rather than needs, autonomy rather than care. The emergence of radical social work in the 1970s and '80s, and its associated techniques of participation and empowerment, similarly opened up spaces for a rights-based approach to social care. Whilst very few service users in our study had access to oppositional discourses, the specialist teams did mobilize an understanding of the social theory of disability in their everyday assessment practice in ways which made them more responsive to people's own risk assessments and strategies. On the hospital team, more traditional social work techniques, notably advocacy, had also survived the industrialization of care.

Culpitt argues that neo-liberal discourses of risk have rendered impotent normative arguments about needs and rights, once used to defend the case for social support (1999: 138). In this chapter we have tried to show that, although dominant modes of risk assessment are central to the bodily welfare order, oppositional discourses of risk not only survive on the front-line of community care but also resonate with claims for human interdependence.

Under a New Labour government, attempts are being made to bring health and social care closer together, through the National Service Frameworks and Health Improvement Programmes for example. Moreover, *Modernising Social Services* sternly warns that: 'Social services must aim wherever possible to help people get better, to improve their health and social functioning rather than just "keep them going"' (DH 1998, para. 2.11). The focus of community care seems set to shift from minimizing dependency by restricting services only to those at greatest risk towards actively promoting independence, ideally through participation in the labour market, but otherwise by providing rehabilitative or preventative support or by encouraging people to manage their own care through direct payments schemes.

What is arguably under way is the reconstruction of community care as a tool of preventative health care, a means of governing the dangerous welfare 'other'. Social relations are no longer determined simply by differential access to key resources, rather corporeal cleavages have opened up as the body is reflexively transformed into a form of 'physical capital', convertible into other types of capital – economic, social, cultural (Falk 1994; Featherstone 1991; Giddens 1992; Shilling 1993). Ablebodiedness has become synonymous with worthiness for consumption, whilst the sick, the disabled and the aged are excluded by norms of youth, athleti-cism and beauty. The risks posed by bodies failing to conform to new standards of health and fitness must be combated by enhancing their capacity for coping independently.

References

Alaszewski, A. (1998) 'Health and welfare: managing risk in late modern society', in A. Alaszewski, L. Harrison and J. Manthorpe (eds) *Risk, Health and Welfare: Policies, strategies and practice*, Buckingham: Open University Press.

Aldridge, M. (1996) 'Dragged to Market: being a profession in the postmodern world', *British Journal of Social Work*, 26(2): 177–94.

Armstrong, D. (1983) *Political anatomy of the body: medical knowledge in Britain in the twentieth century* Cambridge: Cambridge University Press.

—— (1993) 'Public health spaces and the fabrication of identity', *Sociology*, 27(3): 393–404

Audit Commission (1993) *Taking Care: progress with care in the community*, London: HMSO.

Bamford, T. (1990) *The Future of Social Work*, Basingstoke: Macmillan.

Beck, U. (1992) *Risk Society: towards a new modernity*, London: Sage.

Blaxter, M. (1976) *The Meaning of Disability*, London: Heinemann.

Brown, H. and Smith, H. (1993) 'Women Caring for People: the mismatch between rhetoric and reality', *Policy and Politics*, 21(3).

Carter, S. (1995) 'Boundaries of danger and uncertainty: an analysis of the technological culture of risk assessment', in J. Gabe (ed.) *Medicine, Health and Risk: sociological approaches*, Oxford: Blackwell.

Castel, R. (1991) 'From dangerousness to risk', in G. Burchell, C. Gordon and P. Miller (eds) *The Foucault Effect: Studies in Governmentality*, Hemel Hempstead: Harvester Wheatsheaf.

Challis, D. (1992) 'Providing alternatives to long stay hospital care for frail elderly patients: Is it cost effective?', *International Journal of Geriatric Psychiatry*, 7: 773–81.

Cheetham, J. (1993) 'Social work and community care in the 1990s: pitfalls and potential', in R. Page and J. Baldock (eds) *Social Policy Review 5*, Canterbury: Social Policy Association.

Committee on Local Authority and Allied Personal Social Services (1968) *The Seebohm Report*, Cmd 3703, London: HMSO.

Crawford, R. (1984) 'A cultural account of "health": control, release and the social body', in J.B. McKinlay (ed.) *Issues in the Political Economy of Health Care*, London: Tavistock.

Culpitt, I. (1999) *Social Policy and Risk*, London: Sage.

Davis, A., Ellis, K. and Rummery, K. (1997) *Access to Assessment: perspectives of practitioners, disabled people and carers*, Bristol: The Policy Press.

Davis, L. (1995) *Enforcing Normalcy: Disability, deafness, and the body*, London: Verso.

Department of Health (DH) (1989) *Caring for People*, Cmd 849, London: HMSO.

—— (1998) *Modernising Social Services: Promoting independence, improving protection, raising standards*, Cm 4169, London: HMSO.

Dominelli, L. (1996) 'Deprofessionalising Social Work: anti-oppressive practice, competences and postmodernism', *British Journal of Social Work*, 26(2): 153–75.

Donzelot, J. (1979) *The Policing of Families: welfare versus the state*, London: Hutchinson.

Douglas, M. (1990) 'Risk as a forensic resource', *Daedalus*, 119(4): 1–16.

Ellis, K. (1993) *Squaring the Circle: user and carer participation in needs assessment*, York: Joseph Rowntree Foundation/Community Care.

—— (1999a) 'Welfare and Bodily Order: Theorising Transitions in Corporeal Discourse', in K. Ellis and H. Dean (eds) *Social Policy and the Body: transitions in corporeal discourse*, Basingstoke: Macmillan.

—— (1999b) 'The Care of the Body', in K. Ellis and H. Dean (eds) *Social Policy and the Body: transitions in corporeal discourse*, Basingstoke: Macmillan.

—— Davis, A. and Rummery, K. (1999) 'Needs Assessment, Street-level Bureaucracy and the New Community Care', *Social Policy and Administration*, 33(3): 262–80.

Falk, P. (1994) *The Consuming Body*, London: Sage.

Featherstone, M. (1991) 'The Body in Consumer Culture', in M. Featherstone, M. Hepworth and B. Turner (eds) *The Body, Social Process and Cultural Theory*, London: Sage.

Foucault, M. (1979) *Discipline and Punish*, Harmondsworth: Penguin.

Giddens, A. (1991) *Modernity and Self-Identity: self and society in the late modern age*, Cambridge: Polity Press.

—— (1992) *The Transformation of Intimacy: sexuality, love and eroticism in modern societies*, Cambridge: Polity Press.

—— (1994) *Beyond Left and Right: the future of radical politics*, Cambridge: Polity Press.

Hadley, R. and Clough, R. (1996) *Care in Chaos: frustration and challenge in community care*, London: Cassell.

Hewitt, M. (1991) 'Bio-politics and social policy: Foucault's account of welfare', in M. Featherstone, M. Hepworth and B. S. Turner (eds.) *The Body: Social Process and Cultural Theory*, London: Sage.

Hill, M. and Bramley, G. (1986) *Analysing Social Policy*, Oxford: Martin Robertson.

Hughes, B. (1995) *Older People and Community Care: critical theory and practice*, Buckingham: Open University Press.

Hughes, B. and Mtezuka, E.M. (1992) 'Social work and older women', in M. Langan and L. Day (eds) *Women, oppression and social work*, London: Routledge and Kegan Paul.

Hugman, R. (1994) 'Social work and Case Management in the UK: models of professionalism and elderly people', *Ageing and Society*, 14(3): 237–53.

Langan, M. and Clarke, J. (1994) 'Managing in the Mixed Economy of Care', in J. Clarke, A. Cochrane and E. McLaughlin (eds) *Managing Social Policy*, London: Sage.

Lawson, J. (1996) 'A framework of risk assessment and management for older people', in H. Kemshall and J. Pritchard (eds.) *Good Practice in Risk Assessment and Risk Management*, London: Jessica Kingsley.

Levick, P. (1992) 'The janus face of community care legislation: an opportunity for radical possibilities', *Critical Social Policy*, 12(1).

Lewis, J. and Glennerster, H. (1996) *Implementing the new community care*, Buckingham: Open University Press.

Lupton, D. (1994) *Medicine as Culture. Illness, disease and the body in Western societies*, London: Sage.

Means, R. (1995) 'Older people and the personal social services', in D. Gladstone (ed.) *British Social Welfare: past, present and future*, London: UCL Press.

Newman, J. and Clarke, J. (1994) 'Going about our business? The managerialisation of public services', in J. Clarke, A. Cochrane and E. McLaughlin (eds) *Managing Social Policy*, London: Sage.

Petersen, A. (1997) 'Risk, governance and the new public health', in A. Petersen and R. Bunton (eds) *Foucault, Health and Medicine*, London: Routledge.

Reed, J. (1998) 'Care and protection for older people', in B. Heyman (ed.) *Risk, Health and Health Care: A Qualitative Approach*, London: Arnold.

Rose, N. (1993) 'Government, authority and expertise in advanced liberalism', *Economy and Society*, 22(3): 283–99.

Sainsbury, S. (1995) 'Disabled people and the personal social services', in D. Gladstone (ed.) *British Social Welfare Past, present and future*, London: UCL Press.

Schatzki, T.R. and Natter, W. (eds) (1996) *The Social and Political Body*, New York: The Guildford Press.

Shilling, C. (1993) *The Body and Social Theory*, London: Sage.

Smith, G. (1980) *Social need: policy, practice and research*, London: Routledge and Kegan Paul.

Social Services Inspectorate (1991) *Care Management and Assessment: practitioners' guide*, London: HMSO.

Thane, P. (1982) *The Foundations of the Welfare State*, London: Longman.

Titmuss, R. (1963) *Essays on the Welfare State*, second edition, London: Allen and Unwin.

Turner, B. (1996) *The Body and Society*, second edition, London: Sage.

Twigg, J. and Atkin, K. (1994) *Carers Perceived: policy and practice in informal care*, Buckingham: Open University Press.

Webb, A. and Wistow, G. (1987) *Social Work, Social Care and Social Planning: the personal social services since Seebohm*, Harlow: Longman.

Williams, F. (1989) *Social Policy: a critical introduction*, Cambridge: Polity Press.

Williams, S.J. and Bendelow, G. (1998) *The Lived Body: Sociological themes, embodied issues*, London: Routledge.

Chapter 10

Social insecurity and the informal economy

Survival strategies on a South London estate

David Smith and John Macnicol

The economic transformations that have affected Britain and other industrialized economies over the past twenty-five years have changed the labour market prospects of many citizens. Increasingly, low-paid work – often part-time, service-based and insecure – is replacing the 'traditional', blue-collar work offerings of 'organized' capitalism. An adjunct to this has been the growth of a socially and economically marginalized group at the bottom of society. Neither the terms 'underclass' nor 'social exclusion' effectively capture the complex mix of economic, social and demographic forces that have combined to fashion this new social problem. For example, the government's current social exclusion initiatives tend to concentrate upon very obvious symptoms of marginality – teenage pregnancy, lone parenthood, benefit dependency, anti-social behaviour, school exclusions, rough sleeping – rather than the structural economic forces that are worsening prospects for those at the bottom of society. As such, the perspective of the Cabinet Social Exclusion Unit is questionable. For example, Ruth Levitas has criticized the Blairite 'social integrationist' version of social exclusion as fetishizing paid work, neglecting the importance of unpaid work and ignoring wider structural inequalities: by this process, she observes, 'attention is drawn away from the inequalities and differences among the included' (Levitas 1998: 7; see also Byrne 1999).

In this chapter, we examine the low paid, the casually employed and participants in the informal labour market – the classic working poor, who do not normally fall under the rubric of 'social exclusion'. The area upon which the research is based is a large inter-war housing estate spanning two boroughs, Merton and Sutton, on the fringes of South London/Surrey, built by the London County Council to relieve overcrowding in Inner London; it houses around 40,000 residents, roughly split between owner-occupiers and council tenants. We will focus on the 'survival strategies' adopted by the residents, who are seeking to come to terms with a changing labour market which is at the cutting edge of the new post-industrial economy. Within the constraints imposed upon them by highly localized economic conditions, they *do* work hard – often articulating strong work-ethic sentiments and convincingly refuting the suggestion that more 'work obligation' should be applied to the poor (Mead 1986, 1992). But, as will be shown, the work they perform is often fragmented, unpredictable and uncertain.

The term 'survival strategies' may be rather redolent of 1960s 'street life' studies and can sometimes imply a naive romanticization of poverty; but it nevertheless serves a useful purpose, providing one bears in mind Bill Jordan's observation that 'strategies' pursued at an individual or household level are themselves set by 'strategies' pursued at a higher level by collective actors such as the state, corporations and other institutions (Jordan *et al.* 1992; Jordan 1996). Recent sociological explorations of risk are also relevant. In its first incarnation, risk theory was applied rather generally, to globalization, new labour market structures and the concomitant uncertainties of postmodernity (Giddens 1994); its most successful particular application was to ecological issues (Beck 1992). However, recent discussions have broadened in scope: hence Beck includes 'underemployment' in his five interlinked processes that constitute 'second modernity' (Beck 1999: 2). There have been some successful attempts to break away from the rather elitist implications of risk theory, and apply it more specifically to social policy (Culpitt 1999). In particular, its models of rationality, with human beings as reflexive agents, have much potential for application at ground level (Taylor-Gooby 2000). In this chapter, we propose to explore the strategies deployed by the residents of one housing estate, not only in terms of ways of obtaining a minimum income, but also by reference to the values and identities held by them: for example, how do they construct narratives to explain what has happened to their economic environment within a generation, does a strong work ethic still prevail, what range of 'choices' are open to them and do they themselves espouse the idea of 'social exclusion'? We will focus upon those who hover between income from state benefits and income from the informal labour market (often combining the two). Just how do ordinary people cope with the new risks and insecurities engendered by a major economic transformation?

From the global to the local: economic and labour market change in Merton/Sutton 1981–99

In Britain and the USA over the past two decades, one consequence of the realities of the 'global economy' has been the retreat of the state from economic and social intervention as a strategy to stimulate market-led growth and the development of a 'flexible labour market', assisted by deregulation, privatization and organizational 'de-layering'. This has led to an increased reliance on 'outsourcing', subcontract-ing, self-employment and small business growth, resulting in both 'core' and 'periphery' firms. Central to the development of a 'flexible' labour market has been the distinction between 'functionally' and 'numerically' flexible workers (Atkinson 1984). The former comprise the nucleus of the firm, the 'core' of multi-skilled workers holding full-time, relatively well paid and secure employment. The latter are either employed largely under conditions of insecurity (which is built into the structure of an increasingly precarious formal employment regime) (Allen and Henry 1995), or occupy part-time, temporary or casualized jobs – in effect, a 'reserve army' of labour to be utilized as and when required in the volatile and competitive environment of today's labour market. As Kumar notes, this phenomenon is most advanced, not in 'leading edge' manufacturing firms, but in service industries and the public sector (Kumar 1995). These labour market changes have brought about profound alterations in individual consciousness and behaviour as citizens have been removed from familiar and traditional cultural patterns (Beck 1992). There has also been a promotion of a more intensive differentiation of class positions as the class structure becomes increasingly diversified and a pattern of inequality based upon access to extensive and increasingly privatized consumption rather than production emerges (Saunders 1989: 309–42; Crook *et al*. 1992: 121).

Several problems arise in attempting to define the 'local labour market', as the region under study here comprises a network of overlapping sub-markets interacting strongly with each other (Buck *et al*. 1986). However, for the low-paid, unskilled, part-time workers and for women with family commitments, labour market opportunities may be highly localized, and the fortunes of individuals and households tied more closely to the expansion and decline of opportunities within their immediate locality. Economic changes in both boroughs through the 1980s and 1990s reflected changes occurring at both national and regional levels, with employment patterns shifting away from manufacturing and towards the service sector. Merton, an important site for the development of 'new industries' (consumer and electrical goods) in the 1920s and 1930s, had a manufacturing sector that accounted for 36.3 per cent of employment in the borough in 1981. By 1996, as a result of plant closures and relocation, this had fallen to 15.1 per cent of total employment (London Research Centre 1999).

Growth areas indicate an increasing polarization of employment opportunities, as the expanding banking, finance and public administration sectors have increased the supply of managerial and professional opportunities (London Borough of Merton 1994). At the same time, there has been a large growth of low-wage employment in retail, catering and hotels, and in 'personal services', as the demand for skilled and semi-skilled manual workers has contracted. These trends have been accompanied by a notable restructuring of the balance between full-time and part-time work, and between men and women. Both boroughs have experienced a decline in full-time male employment and a growth in full-time female employment. In Merton, full-time male employment fell from 50.4 per cent to 45.3 per cent of the total workforce between 1991 and 1997, while for women such employment grew from 21.8 per cent to 25.0 per cent over the same period. In Sutton, female full-time employment grew from 30.3 per cent to 35.1 per cent of the total workforce over the same period; by contrast, full-time male employment declined from 43.2 per cent to 39.5 per cent (London Research Centre 1999). This is projected to decline further to 28.6 per cent by 2006 (Employment Service 1998). These changes have reflected the pattern of economic decline and renewal, the latter mainly occurring in those areas that employ high proportions of largely female, low-grade service sector employees. It is those areas that have experienced the most rapid job growth in the boroughs – retail, catering, hotels and 'personal services' – that contain the highest proportion of Britain's 1,900,000 to 2,400,000 employees aged over 18 who, in 1998, were earning less than the national minimum wage (Wilkinson 1998).

The area has also experienced a growth in small business formation and in self-employment, the fostering of which has been identified as a key objective in the boroughs' economic regeneration strategies (London Borough of Sutton 1997). The growth of self-employment has often been heralded as highlighting the centrality of the market and entrepreneurial values. Less optimistic accounts emphasize a growing informalization on the margins of the formal/informal economies, the erosion of the institutional power of organized labour and growing convergence between the labour market structures of the 'advanced' and 'developing' worlds (Castells and Portes 1989). Evidence also points to growing differences in income and a growth of 'low income' self-employed, who in the 1990s claimed in-work benefits such as Family Credit. A key element in recent welfare reforms has been an increasing acceptance of the use of such benefits, thus increasing flexibility and competitiveness by depressing wages further and allowing the market to respond by creating more low-wage labour (Eardley and Cordon 1996; Grove and Stewart 1999).

From interviews with several people involved in very small business enterprises in the area, it can be seen that a 'flexible' pool of labour is a key resource in the early years of a business. As one small employer explained:

> I wouldn't survive unless I cut corners . . . you've got cab offices competing with taxis, Indian restaurants competing with pizza shops, wine bars competing against pubs. You've got small shops competing against big shops and if we didn't use them [cash workers] we'd go under.

The introduction of minimum wage and employment legislation is likely to accelerate the trend towards self-employment as firms attempt to gain a competitive advantage and free themselves from any obligation to the employee (Jordan and Travers 1998). As one respondent, working for a small cleaning contractor, said:

> Small businesses rely on people like us to tide them over until they can be completely above board. How else can they get to that level? They get around it like A: if anybody comes for a job and they're not dodgy, she says to them, 'You have to be self employed and you can sort out your own tax and national insurance'. Then it's not down to her.

The estate

The larger part of the estate is situated in the Borough of Sutton, which was profiled in the 1998 Department of the Environment, Transport and the Regions Index of Local Deprivation as the least deprived borough in London with an official unemployment rate of 3.7 per cent (compared to 6.7 per cent for Greater London) and some 20 per cent of its wards among the wealthiest 10 per cent in England. Analysis at the borough level, however, disguises large variations between areas of prosperity and decline: in June 1996 unemployment rates across the three wards in the estate averaged 13 per cent, largely concentrated among males in the 25–34 and 35–44 age brackets, who constitute some 65 per cent of unemployed on the estate (London Borough of Sutton 1996). The locality also has a considerably higher rate of long-term unemployment than the borough as a whole, and has witnessed a decline in economic activity since the early 1980s. In 1981, 55.5 per cent of the resident population of working age were economically active, falling to 42.5 per cent by 1991, despite a shift during the same period towards a younger age structure with a rise in young families with children. There has also been an increase in lone parents on the estate, from 2.0 per cent of households in 1981 to 13.5 per cent in 1991 – over double the borough average (London Borough of Sutton 1981 and 1991).

What these data point to is the spatial significance of restructuring, suggesting that these processes impact unevenly on different localities and on different households within them. This primarily reflects the socio-economic characteristics of those housed in social housing, consisting of residential concentrations of groups in a weak competitive position in the labour market. The spatial significance of restructuring was encapsulated in Wilson's concept of 'social isolation', which has come in for some criticism – not least for its perpetuation of the 'ecological fallacy' (the attribution of a shared cultural outlook among individuals sharing the same spatial location) (Wilson 1987: 60–2). In response, Byrne observes that this stems from viewing class as an individual rather than a collective phenomenon and that:

> From any sociological perspective it makes sense to consider effects at the neighbourhood level as of potential significance in the formation of collectivities. We have to think in spatial terms precisely because of the crucial significance of spatial segregation in the formation of bases of social action. . . . We need to see if there are spatial concentrations of deprived neighbourhoods and to examine the nature of deprivation and exclusion from work within them.
>
> (Byrne 1995: 99)

Networks, social capital and inclusion

Previous sections have examined the processes that have assisted a move towards increasing informalization and flexibility in the lower reaches of the labour market within the local context. They contextualize the issues to be addressed and should serve as a precursor to a qualitative study of the ways in which economic changes have altered the framework of opportunities facing individuals and households and of how these individuals and households have experienced and responded to changes in their labour market location. Quantitative data may be underlaid by a wide variety of cultural designs for living and may thus explain little about the interplay between structural constraints, individual agency and the social relations in which economic life is situated.

The data presented here are drawn from an ESRC-funded ethnographic study based on the estate and the surrounding area. This has involved participant observation, qualitative interviews and the collection of work-histories with a sample of thirty-five residents located to a greater or lesser extent on the margins between low wage, short-term and insecure formal employment, benefit dependency and various sources of undeclared income. A further thirty interviews were conducted with participants in local employment training and New Deal schemes, with unemployed residents and with the low paid in receipt of in-work benefits.

The sample has been constructed using a 'snowball' or 'chain referral' method. Although the methodological issues raised by such an approach cannot be pursued here, Coleman has noted that it is uniquely designed for sociological research since it allows for sampling of natural interactional units (Coleman 1958). The ability to use relevant knowledge of the area and pre-existing contacts has proved advantageous in locating informants with knowledge and experience of informal work. While the use of such methods justifiably raises objections regarding the representativeness of the sample and the extent of the 'income generating' methods or lifestyles described, which will remain undetectable through such methods, it also provides more valid data through allowing the possibility of what Glaser and Strauss have referred to as 'theoretical sampling' – that is, targeting those with knowledge of a particular area of the social world – and may be the only feasible method for sampling 'hidden populations' (Glaser and Strauss 1967; Lee 1993).

More importantly, the social relations underpinning snowball sampling tend to promote a sample similar in its attributes. Such a homogeneous population may prove beneficial in exploring the nature of social networks (how the individual uses them in generating employment and the jobs that informal methods provide). Morris, for example, suggests that broken employment is closely related to the jobs available through informal support networks due to the social contacts that form around insecure employment and ultimately do much to reproduce the system (Morris 1995: 69).

Several field studies have stressed the degree to which economic behaviour is related to social processes influenced through personal relations to kin and friends and the role of networks of such relations in circulating 'social capital' (Kelly 1994). Although not the major source of work, information on jobs provided through personal contacts, via locally based subcontractors, provided an important supply of work opportunities for many of the respondents. The trend towards subcontracting has made informal recruitment through networks of the unemployed an important tactic for a small employer seeking greater flexibility (MacDonald 1994). For example, during the course of the fieldwork, interviews have been conducted with several cleaners, couriers, caterers and gardeners servicing some of the large office developments and institutions in the area who are employed and recruited under such circumstances. Employed by informal family-type firms or locally-based small contractors, they represent the low wage, casualized end of tiered layers of subcontracting.

Although word-of-mouth recruitment has existed throughout the industrial era (Pahl 1984), Sassen views the increasing prominence of the informal sector and shift towards more informal recruitment methods as closely tied to the process of tertiarization. The high growth sectors generate a large amount of low-wage, casualized work, both directly, through the occupational structure of these sectors, and indirectly, through the ancillary sector and consumption practices of the new, high-income service class. At the same time, a growing informal sector emerges that services the needs of the corporate economy: office cleaners, messengers, delivery staff, baby-minders and domestic cleaners (Sassen 1990, esp. 245–318; Gorz 1989: 5). In other words, the affluent households in the area provide abundant opportunities for informal work. As one interviewee testified,

> You've got a lot of career women round here and while they're out chasing their careers who do you think's ironing their blouses and looking after their kids?

Access to employment, formal or informal, is largely contingent on an individual's contacts and, crucially, the extent to which a network is composed of persons themselves playing multiple roles in several fields as captured by Granovetter's notion of 'strong' and 'weak' ties (Granovetter 1985). For example, several respondents have indicated a close interrelationship and fluidity between formal, informal and more illegal income-generating methods as the contacts and information tapped in one sphere can be utilized to increase social capital and enhance opportunities in another. One respondent remarked that the web of contacts established during a spell of low-level drug dealing have been crucial in providing access to cash work:

> It's [cash work] easy to get, really, just by asking about. If you've either got a lot of friends working cash-in-hand jobs or know a wide circle of people then you'll always find something. . . . We got to know a wide circle of people through dealing, and, alright, the majority of them were tossers, but you always get to know people that are handy in some way or another; we know a lot of people involved in it, running little businesses and that, so I don't have to look too hard.

The emphasis given to cash work as a 'survival strategy' for downgraded manual workers often overlooks the fact that it encompasses a wide range of activities, and thereby parallels the formal economy in another important respect: access to the form of work is dependent on previous skills and work experience (Pahl 1984). The personal relations on which these opportunities are based give a cumulative advantage to those in certain networks and exclude others seeking alternative sources of income. Another respondent working undeclared for a site clearance contractor explained how these recruitment methods operate – resulting in a 'core' and 'periphery' workforce akin to developments said to be transforming the formal labour market (Williams and Windebank 1998).

> That's how it works with G.T. [builders]. He's got his regular crew that's three or four blokes that he'll give work to near enough fulltime. Then when he needs extra there's about five like me that he'll call when he's busy. He knows we're alright because it's one of the regulars that put us onto him, so it's OK, and that's how it works with G.T. If you're in you're in, but if you're no good you're down the road.

For skilled workers – mechanics and tradesmen among this sample for instance – working 'off the cards' can bring a regular income higher than would be obtainable under more formal work relations, more autonomy and freedom from bureaucratic hassles. The theme of autonomy recurred frequently among all cash workers regardless of the type of work they were involved in. For example, at the more successful end of the sample a car dealer/mechanic whose business is largely based on the estate and surrounding area explained the benefits of staying outside the formal system in the following terms:

> I think it's having to get involved in tax, paperwork – all that'd mean learning to do it myself or paying someone to do it and it's the overheads . . . it's, like, a nice idea, but I'm raking in enough as it is and in the end you've got to ask yourself, 'would I be much better off?'. I'm quite happy with my life as it is: I do alright, do work that I enjoy. That's more than you can say for a lot of people round here.

For the majority of the sample, however, cash work is often highly irregular, fluctuating between bouts of usually low-paid, short-term employment and the search for further opportunities. Hence the ability to manipulate past contacts forged in the formal, informal or illegal (usually drug-based) economies, and a willingness to move between these spheres as and when opportunities arise, is vital to securing a regular income outside the boundaries of formal employment. For another respondent, formal employment in a timber yard provided the original outlet for his small-scale drug dealing over the counter to incoming tradesmen, which then provided a source for cash work once the formal employment had ended:

> Through my time at the timber yard I got to know loads of builders and I used to sell a lot of draw on sites so I got to know loads of them, like loads of them have been regular customers for years now and if they need a hand they'll just call my mobile and say 'what are you doing next week?'.

Fieldwork among this extended network reveals that it not only provides information and access to work. Of greater importance in maintaining an acceptable standard of living is the role of the network in providing multiple channels for the supply, distribution and information relating to cheap goods and services. This develops into a vast underground-trading network that transcends the boundaries of the estate to include the adjacent area and neighbouring estates. Demand is sustained by the opportunity to acquire goods that would normally be out of the reach of many residents. This aspect of informal exchange frequently crosses legal boundaries, providing a ready market for stolen and counterfeit goods supplied largely by local drug addicts, and is rationalized in economic terms and in terms of acquiring a lifestyle – measured by ownership of certain consumer items – comparable to others in the community (cf. Parker *et al*. 1988: 105–8). As the lone parent working full-time explained,

> My little boy, now he's at the age where he wants Nike and Adidas, and so do I, and I can't afford to buy them for both of us, so if anything comes up cheap, I'll take it straight away.

Lifecourse transitions, employment insecurity and the social context of exclusion

Perceptions about the relation between formal employment, benefits and undeclared work are shaped by a combination of several factors. In an area of low unemployment and high job growth the complaint is not about the lack of work so much as the lack of legitimate opportunities to attain a reasonable standard of living from the jobs on offer. The areas of job growth are commonly viewed as not designed to pay a 'family wage', and are no longer an option at the major transitions that mark the passage to adulthood (leaving home and/or the birth of a child):

> When I was at home I'd take anything because even if the money was crap I'd give my Mum a bit and I'd still have eighty quid or so, and this was pocket money: I had nothing to pay for. When you leave home and have kids and that, it's a whole different ball game: you can't take those crap jobs any more because they're designed for kids or women.

As Jordan *et al.* found in a study of a housing estate in Exeter, the reduction in formal work opportunities has been partly offset by an expansion of casualized, unskilled work which, linked to the growth of meanstested benefits, has combined to produce a culture of undeclared work (Jordan *et al.* 1992: 122–5). Many, when discussing lifecourse transitions, mentioned the reappraisal of their labour market location that accompanies such transitions:

> What changed things for me totally was that when I moved onto the estate I had my own home to provide for . . . so I worked out at the time that I'd have to be earning quite a large sum of money to live to a certain standard.

Even if I was earning £250 a week – and where am I going to earn that sort of money? – I wouldn't be much better off, and the option of earning more money and having my main overheads covered just became more viable at the time.

Calculating the earnings from her current undeclared job (house-cleaning for a small contractor), on top of her benefit allowance, one respondent estimates that she earns a disposable income of around £140 per week for herself and her daughter, unrealistic in the formal labour market even with the marginal gains of in-work benefits. Assessments of the opportunities available in the formal labour market are grounded in the respondents' own experiences and in the experiences of the 'working poor' who live in the same locality. Several mentioned being considerably better off financially than friends and family in low paid formal employment:

What can a woman earn if she's on her own and got to be back by 3 o'clock? A part-time job's all she can do and it's never going to be enough, so you're forced to take different routes. . . . They say that if you go to work in a shit job they'll still pay some of your rent and you won't be worse off. No you won't, but you won't be better off; and at the end of the day why should you have to leave your kid all day with someone else for no reason?

These issues are relevant to a clearer appreciation of social exclusion as experienced and understood in its social context, particularly regarding its current popularity in political and policy discourse where it tends to be equated with exclusion from the formal labour market. Those who are excluded from the formal labour market are more likely to describe their situation in terms of older notions of relative poverty and the prevailing consumption practices of the surrounding community. All had a clear notion of what a 'decent wage' should be – around £250 per week net being the consensus – and all were adamant that combining various forms of undeclared income underpinned by the benefit system was the only feasible way to achieve it.

Nevertheless, while economic calculations play a central role in influencing behaviour, they are also affected by other social and psychological considerations. Howe notes that 'unemployment is a great financial, social and psychological burden, but so too is work when it is low paid and has to be endured for long hours and in bad conditions' (Howe 1990: 85). The growth of low paid, insecure and menial jobs, in combination with increasing state surveillance and coercion to take such jobs, and, more importantly, to remain in them under the threat of forfeiting access to the benefit system, has combined to intensify the precariousness and insecurity of those at the lower end of the labour market, and make undeclared work backed up by benefits an increasingly logical option in securing a regular income and modicum of security.[1] The real fear frequently voiced is not of the loss of income support, which can be recuperated from cash work anyway, but of losing access to housing benefit. This engenders considerable anxiety. As one respondent explained:

> I'm scared to give up the social, and it's not so much the money it's the rent and that's a lot of people's worry, because once you're getting your rent paid it'd be awful if they stopped it, and that's why I won't sign off. Because if I can't manage my rent I'll be evicted.

In this sense, although cash work is similar to formal work in regard to its nature and levels of pay, it is constructed as preferable because it provides more options to leave, since the benefit system provides a base of security while the availability of cash work ensures that another job will come along:

> I'm scared that they'll phone me up and stick me on a till at Tesco's for £4 an hour. At least at the moment I'm free to take it or leave it. There's only so long you can do those sorts of jobs because they do your head in . . . I mean, with what I'm doing now at least I can jack it in if I get too fed up and something else always comes along. If I upped and walked out of Tesco's they wouldn't pay my income support and rent and I'd be stuck. I'd have no choice because you can't jack it in when you've got rent and the rest to pay, so you're trapped.

Suttles described how, in low income neighbourhoods, practical morality takes precedence over abstract morality, implying that material conditions in the lower class may be more powerful in shaping behaviour and values than in other social classes (Suttles 1968: 231–2). Benefit fraud was justified as legitimate in providing an adequate lifestyle for individuals and families within a context of restricted options; far from devaluing the work ethic, it instead provided an essential foundation to irregular and low pay (see Dean 1996). When seen from the insider's viewpoint, the strategies deployed appear less as evidence of a 'welfare dependent underclass', and more as a way of *avoiding* 'underclass' status, as understood by those for whom such a status remains a constant and nagging possibility, comprising dire poverty, exclusion from work, exclusion from the networks that provide access to work and exclusion from the status symbols that denote distance from this ever-present underclass. In the social relations of the estate it is the genuinely unemployed who are designated as the real underclass and often castigated for their inability or reluctance to participate in the burgeoning cash economy:[2]

> You can tell the real people on income support because they're really raggedy and scruffy, blankets for curtains and all that . . . I don't know why they don't work . . . well, they're usually impaired in some way, so maybe they're not in the market for work, or else they don't believe in it, which is a bad attitude if you've got kids: if I lived with my parents and had a cash-in-hand job it'd be unthinkable of me to sign on as well but now it's different.

The development of workfare programmes and in-work benefits has been presented as a means of institutionalizing the low-paid casualized work often undertaken in the informal economy. The views of the low paid, the unemployed and those combining cash work with benefits among this sample all suggest that social exclusion cannot be tackled by coercing them into a low-wage, 'flexible' labour market. The findings presented here suggest that those participating in the cash economy have few incentives to participate in formal work, since what is offered is mostly viewed with extreme scepticism, while the possibility that taking an entry-level job will lead to a better future seems uncertain compared to the relative security and immediate advantages of the cash economy:

> £3-something minimum wage. . . . I said 'thanks Tone' and I voted for him! It's easy to talk about scroungers when you're on fifty grand a year. It's not like 40 quid a day on site plus dole is the best you can get, and this fraud crackdown won't make any difference because there's a big gap between doing alright and not doing alright, and you can't do alright these days with what's in the job centres.

Conclusion

This chapter has tried to examine the responses of ordinary people to the growing economic insecurities and risks created by post-industrial capitalism. Several themes have been emphasized. A strong work ethic still prevails, but it has become adapted to a new economic order in which (as in the nineteenth-century labour market) the distinctions between 'formal' and 'informal' work are becoming blurred. Supporting oneself and one's family is still a mark of honour, and this is increasingly being achieved by juggling a combination of sources – cash-in-hand work in the informal economy, casual or part-time semi-formal work, and reciprocal services in kind, often underpinned by benefit claiming. Indeed, conventional categorical benefits are increasingly being seen as useful in-work benefits: in effect, the residents of the estate are forging their own citizen's income scheme. Many of them have a clear idea of a desirable minimum income level (around £250 per week being the consensus), and the economic 'survival strategy' is to achieve this. Working in the formal economy is often seen as positively disadvantageous, since it involves a loss of personal autonomy and locks one in to rigid structures that are subject to close surveillance by the state.

We have tried, albeit briefly, to examine 'from below' responses not only in terms of 'getting' a living, but also in terms of shared values. Here it is clear that the most of the local residents do not see themselves as 'socially excluded' since they use each other as reference groups. As in the 'depressed areas' of that last period of enormous economic transformation – the 1930s – a community finds itself in a shared economic situation (Runciman 1966: 63–77). It is clear that residents try hard to support themselves and their families within the tight constraints of local economic conditions, combining different sources of income and making intelligent choices – within a restricted range of available options – about the division between each. All in all, the picture from this estate is one of creativity and resilience in dealing with the impact of a new industrial revolution.

Acknowledgements

The research upon which this chapter is based is funded by the ESRC (award no. R00429734632).

Notes

1 Borgois, discussing the psychological and cultural aspects of the new service employment, refers to the 'cultural dislocations of the new service economy', arguing that obedience to the norms of this economy are in direct contrast to street culture's definitions of personal dignity: 'Their macho-proletarian dream of working an eight-hour shift plus overtime throughout their adult lives has been replaced by the nightmare of poorly paid, highly feminised, office-support service work' (Borgois 1995: 141).
2 See Howe (1994) for a relevant discussion of the role of ideological discourses of unemployment among a working class community of Belfast.

References

Allen, J. and Henry, N. (1995) 'Fragments of industry and employment: contract service work and the shift towards precarious employment', in R. Crompton, D. Gallie, and D. Purcell (eds) *Changing Forms of Employment – Organisations, Skills and Gender*, London: Routledge.

Atkinson, J. (1984) 'Manpower strategies for flexible organisations', *Personnel Management*, 16, August, 28–31.

Beck, U. (1992) *Risk Society: Towards A New Modernity*, London: Sage.

—— (1999) *World Risk Society*, Cambridge: Polity Press.

Borgois, P. (1995) *In Search of Respect: Selling Crack in El Barrio*, New York: Cambridge University Press.

Buck, N., Gordon, I., and Young, K. (1986) *The London Employment Problem*, Oxford: Clarendon Press.

Byrne, D. (1995) 'Deindustrialisation and dispossession: an examination of social division in the industrial city', *Sociology*, 29(1): 98–109.

—— (1999) *Social Exclusion*, Buckingham: Open University Press.

Castells, M. and Portes, C. (1989) 'The origins, dynamics and effects of the informal economy', in A. Portes, M. Castells and L. Benton (eds) *The Informal Economy: Studies in Advanced and Less Developed Countries*, London: Johns Hopkins Press.

Coleman, J.S. (1958) 'Relational analysis: the study of social organisations with survey methods', *Human Organisation* 17, 46–71.

Crook, S., Pakulski, J., Waters, M. (1992) *Postmodernization: Change in Advanced Societies*, London: Sage.

Culpitt, I. (1999) *Social Policy and Risk*, London: Sage.

Dean, H. (1996) 'Unravelling citizenship: the significance of social security benefit fraud', *Critical Social Policy*, 16(3): 3–31.

Eardley, T. and Cordon, A. (1996) *Low Income Self-Employment, Work Benefits and Living Standards: Studies in Cash and Care*, Aldershot: Avebury.

Employment Service, South West London Training and Enterprise Council and South London Training and Enterprise Council (1998) *New Deal Delivery Plan: Sutton, Epsom and Esher District*.

Giddens, A. (1994) *Beyond Left and Right*, Cambridge: Polity Press.

Glaser, B. and Strauss, A. (1967) *The Discovery of Grounded Theory*, Chicago: Aldine.

Gorz, A. (1989) *A Critique of Economic Reason*, London: Verso.

Granovetter, M. (1985) 'Economic action and social structure: the problem of embeddedness', *American Journal of Sociology*, 91(3): 481–510.

Grove, C. and Stewart, J. (1999) 'Market workfare: social security, social regulation and competitiveness', *Journal of Social Policy* 28(1): 73–97.

Howe, L. (1990) *Being Unemployed in Northern Ireland*, Cambridge: Cambridge University Press.

—— (1994) 'Ideology, domination and unemployment', *Sociological Review*, 42(2): 315–39.

Jordan, B., Simon, J., Kay, H., and Redley, M. (1992) *Trapped in Poverty? Labour Market Decisions in Low Income Households*, London: Routledge.

Jordan, B. (1996) *A Theory of Poverty and Social Exclusion*, Oxford: Polity Press.

Jordan, B. and Travers, A. (1998) 'The informal economy: a case study in unrestrained competition', *Social Policy and Administration* 32(3): 292–306.

Kelly, M. (1994) 'Towanda's triumph: social and cultural capital in the transition to adulthood in the urban ghetto', *International Journal of Urban and Regional Research*, 18(1): 88–111.

Kumar, K. (1995) *From Post Industrial to Post Modern Society*, Oxford: Blackwell.

Lee, R. (1993) *Doing Research on Sensitive Topics*, London: Sage.

Levitas, R. (1998) *The Inclusive Society? Social Exclusion and New Labour*, London: Macmillan.

London Borough of Merton (1994) *The Economic Development Strategy 1992/3*, Economic Development Unit.

London Borough of Sutton (1981) *1981 Census: Ward Profiles, St. Helier North and St. Helier South*.

—— (1991) *1991 Census Facts and Figures: Census Information from Northern Wards*.

—— (1997) *Ward Profiles 1996*: Policy and Planning Unit, Chief Executive's Department.

—— (1999) *Sutton Economic Regeneration Strategy 1998/99*.

London Research Centre (1999) *Annual Employment Survey and Census of Employment*.

MacDonald, R. (1994) 'Fiddly jobs, undeclared working and the something for nothing society', *Work, Employment and Society* 8(4): 507–30.

Mead, L. (1986) *Beyond Entitlement: the Social Obligations of Citizenship*, New York: The Free Press.

—— (1992) *The New Politics of Poverty: the Nonworking Poor in America*, New York: Basic Books.

Morris, L. (1995) *Social Divisions: Economic Decline and Social Structural Change*, King's Lynn: UCL Press.

Pahl, R. (1984) *Divisions of Labour*, Oxford: Blackwell.

Parker, H., Bakx, K. and Newcombe, R. (1988) *Living with Heroin: The Impact of a Drugs 'Epidemic' on an English Community*, Milton Keynes: Open University Press.

Runciman, W.G. (1966) *Relative Deprivation and Social Justice*, London: Routledge.
Sassen, S. (1990) *The Global City: New York, London, Tokyo*, Princeton: Princeton University Press.
Saunders, P. (1989) 'Beyond housing classes: the sociological significance of private property rights in means of consumption', in L. McDowell, P. Sarre and C. Hamnett (eds) *Divided Nation: Social and Cultural Change in Britain*, London: Hodder and Stoughton/Open University Press.
Suttles, G.D. (1968) *The Social Order of the Slum*, Chicago: University of Chicago Press.
Taylor-Gooby, P. (ed.) (2000) *Risk, Trust and Welfare*, Basingstoke: Macmillan.
Wilkinson, D. (1998) 'Who are the low paid?', *Labour Market Trends*, 106(12): 617–22.
Williams, C.C. and Windebank, J. (1998) *Informal Employment in the Advanced Economies: Implications for Work and Welfare*, London: Routledge.
Wilson, W.J. (1987) *The Truly Disadvantaged: the Inner City, the Underclass and Public Policy*, Chicago: University of Chicago Press.

Chapter 11

Social capital and waves of innovation in the risk society

Barbara Jones and Bob Miller

Introduction

The formation of social capital is a crucial topic for both descriptive and analytical social science and for the current UK policy agenda of improving levels of social capital, which we conceptualize as formal and informal social practices, institutions, networks and performances. In this context, we argue that it is therefore worthwhile to investigate the relevance of processes analogous to Schumpeter's 'waves of creative destruction' on the assumption that modern capitalism may be programmed to accelerate the rate at which such waves follow on one another. It is obvious that since Western society has been revolutionized many times in the last centuries, it will be difficult to isolate the effects of this factor. The patterns of work, housing, and commuting, which are currently being disrupted, are themselves historically recent. In any particular locality it is possible to ascribe much of the problematic of social exclusion to more immediate effects of the capitalist cycle of boom and slump or the secular decline of 'traditional' industries. The specific feature of the phenomenon we are attempting to describe is that the lifetime of industrial paradigms is tending to become shorter than the active lifetime of individuals. This may be welcomed by many individuals, and new generations may (or may not) grow up accustomed to the resulting effects. One problem for social policy is that individuals will increasingly have to face more than one significant life transition between entering and finally leaving the labour market. At each of these transitions there is a risk of exclusion. This automatically increases individual insecurity. Each of these transitions, whether successful or unsuccessful for the individual, will also be accompanied by a disruption of patterns of social capital, which are not easily rebuilt. The wider effect then, on society, will be more significant than might be indicated by the number of individuals who fail to make these transitions successfully. The need to concentrate on understanding how social capital networks among adults can be preserved across waves of creative destruction and how the mutual trust, knowledge and community lost in these waves can be regenerated in new contexts, becomes urgent. Concurrently, we also need to investigate situations in which patterns of social capital are preserved or generated in a delocalized form and how this can affect the levels of localized social capital.

We have been led to the questions discussed here by questions arising from our current research, which is concerned with skills and knowledge. We are directly concerned with discovering what are likely to be the most robust 'generic' skills within the 'information society' in order to equip individuals with the ability to move with minimum disruption from job to job and from sector to sector.[1] Smoothing such transitions could reduce the frictions that lead to the attrition of social capital. In the mid-twentieth century industrial developments tended to reduce the levels of exchangeable social capital in communities as there was increasing distance between the skills used in industry and those necessary in households and neighbourhoods. This first came to our attention in terms of the increased need for formal training and the difficulties in building on the skills and prior learning of migrant workers. It became apparent that it also played a role in the difficulty in redeploying workers from the paradigmatic heavy industries when these began to shed labour in the 1970s. The penetration of informational and communicational work and technologies may recreate the possibility of widespread use of work-related skills in other contexts, creating a higher potential for the useful sharing of individual human capital through networks of social capital. We have nevertheless focused here on the dangers to levels of social capital arising from the disruption of spatial patterning which accompany these changes.

Creative destruction

Schumpeter's economic theory is unique in the role that he ascribed to entre-preneurs and in the explanation of growth. In a series of works (Schumpeter 1939, 1961, 1976) he developed the idea that it is only innovation which leads to growth, and that the entrepreneur is to be distinguished from the capitalist as well as from the manager, in that the entrepreneur is that person who develops and realizes new combinations in the economy, whether these are new technical methods, new organisational methods, or new markets, for inputs or final products. All non-usurious interest (productive interest) is due to growth initiated by entrepreneurs and without it the capital market that pulls resources away from consumption and from the financing of traditional economic activities would not exist.

Within this context Schumpeter suggested that the long cycles of the capitalist economy (sometimes called Kondratieff long waves, which he considered to be real phenomena although there is still controversy about whether these are genuinely cyclical in origin) are due to the necessarily cyclical nature of innovation.[2]

Essentially innovations are relatively easy to initiate during the downturn of a cycle when resources are underemployed or unemployed. Some of these inno-vations succeed, creating both openings for further innovations and willingness to finance them. Successful new technologies or products create the need for a whole new infrastructure of suppliers, maintenance, and training, and in the case of innovations in transport and communications create new entrepreneurial possi-bilities by connecting markets which were previously isolated. New technologies and products are rapidly found to have other uses than those originally intended, opening further new markets. This gives rise to the 'boom', which proceeds until additional capital is no longer required by the innovative sector. In the long run this would be because the levels of profit generated by the once innovative sectors are brought back into line with general profit levels, so that they no longer attract additional investment.

These cycles can be mapped onto the appearance of particular technological paradigms, within which a period of revolutionary development of new sources of power supply and new transport technologies accompanied by a flowering of major infrastructural investment is followed by a period of the more gradual improvement of the technology followed by the eventual appearance of others. For our purposes the relevance of the theory is that it proposes an economic explanation for the cyclical rather than gradual supersession of one industrial paradigm, and its associated repertoire of skills and knowledge, by another. If taken seriously it therefore creates an assumption that as long as this cycle is not broken by some external factor, the obsolescence of skills and knowledge will itself be cyclical.

Recently a new school of economics in the general tradition of Schumpeter, known as *endogenous growth theory*, has suggested a different explanatory mechanism for the connection of economic cycles with discrete waves of technological innovation. This explanation suggests that major cycles are associated with specific 'General Purpose Technologies' which require major research, development and infrastructural investment.[3] This theory suggests that the downturn is the period during which this investment is preparatory and unproductive, while the boom occurs when it reaches fruition and begins to be profitable. The differences between these theories are quite significant for economic policy, but both versions of the theory suggest an explanation for the cyclical nature of the replacement of dominant technological infrastructures.

Social capital, individualization and risk

These issues can be related to the wider question of the switch from a society characterized primarily by mechanisms for the distribution of resources, capital and income, to one increasingly characterized by mechanisms for the distribution of risk, as depicted by Beck (1992: 19–50 and 139–150; 2000: 67–91). The unequal distribution of resources has always led to unequal life chances, and economic and political events whether caused by anonymous market or social mechanisms or by the decisions of particular entrepreneurs or managements have had catastrophic effects for many individuals. Within the class-based mass industrial society these effects were themselves group effects and took place against a background of overall advance within which displaced individuals could find a new foothold of participation. The individualization of risk that Beck describes takes place against the background of a disconnection between economic growth and employment growth that Beck sees as first making serious inroads into the fabric of German society in the 1980s but as having begun around 1920 in the USA.[4] This means that failure to acquire the particular kind of skills required by each particular phase of market developments can lead to permanent exclusion from the productivity gains of the wider society. There have always been some economic sectors in which distribution of business risk has been finely distributed, such as the patterns of subcontracting in construction. Risk is now *inter alia* distributed through the processes of education and professional training, which individuals must face no longer simply as a filtering process but as a field of genuine alternative investment decisions.

Another aspect of Beck's portrayal of current developments is that the individual becomes increasingly isolated by the requirements of mobility. This ultimately isolates the individual from all natural ties such as those of the family.[5] At the same time the individual, who cannot rely on the permanence of economic organizations and organizational membership, needs to become more connected through networks. These networks will however themselves tend to become more centred on the work situation and work contacts. There is therefore a tendency for embeddedness, the social capital used and maintained within the economic sphere, to supplant and eat up networks of social capital in the wider society. There is a danger that such networks will no longer function as a 'safety net' where they become overly centred on a particular firm or sector which may experience a general crisis or decline. We shall return to this question in the context of new technologies below. The mechanisms which we attempt to identify here are not alternative explanations to those put forward by Beck 2000 (115–16) but represent further strains on the structures of social capital additional to those caused by the market-driven increase of working and travel time which he identifies as eating into the time available for social action.

In our own research we have noticed that there is a significant problem in the development of company in-house proprietary skills. Some such skills arise as part of the development of the products and processes that constitute the basis of the competitive advantage of market-leading firms. Others arise through the reorganization of firms' product and process systems carried out as part of the introduction of new infrastructures of information and communications technology. Another very significant area of skills formation is the field of franchising, which is largely identified with retail and service trades, where the skills and knowledge of the workers are part of the image which is being sold by franchisers. In all of these areas there arises the problem that the skills in question are not available from public training providers or traded on the labour market but can only be acquired by induction into the organizations concerned. For the individual, the decision to 'invest' in such skills is therefore tied up with estimations of the future of the firms involved. Conversely those who are unemployed or working in lower technology areas have no access to knowledge of these developments.

Human capital and social capital

Social capital is a problematic notion. Physical capital is embodied in machinery, buildings, stocks of goods, and infrastructures such as roads and railways. Human capital is a concept which has arisen by analogy with physical capital. It is taken to comprise the knowledge and skills embodied in human beings. This analogy has arisen because of the possibility of investment in human capital.[6] Individuals, families, firms and governments can make a conscious decision to invest a greater or lesser part of their finite resources in education, training, health and welfare with the specific aim of increasing a 'stock' of knowledge and skills that will be useful in the future. This 'stock' of human capital can be usefully viewed as 'appreciating' or 'depreciating' in value. Some kinds of skills and knowledge are subject to variation in supply and demand. Others become obsolete or are subject to intrinsic processes of decay. Some are dependent on use in combination with other skills or other resources. Whether valued in terms of the labour market or in the more intangible terms of other life chances, investment of real economic resources in developing 'human capital' can be subjected to some level of rational calculation and measurement.

In this context, 'social capital' would seem to initially have been a further development of the concept of 'human capital', but one that is even more difficult to measure.[7] When understood in this way, social capital may be defined as that part of the process of accessing the human capital of others that is left out of the mechanisms of the market and the bureaucratized services of the state. Social capital becomes a residual concept, akin to the 'natural economy' and the 'informal economy'. Its area of application is also seen to largely overlap with that sphere which some theorists call 'civil society' in explicit contra-distinction to both the market and the state. This does not necessarily mean that the 'market' and the 'state' as spheres can be completely identified with the laws of the market and the rules of bureaucratic procedures. In fact neither of these mechanisms could operate without informal connections that parallel those seen more openly operating in 'civil society'. It is therefore possible to conceptualize 'social capital' as a reduced and naked form of the same phenomenon that oils the formal mechanisms of the market and the state. Within and between organizations there are informal connections between individuals that parallel those usually seen as constituting 'social capital' when they take place between individuals.[8] Here we will, nevertheless, continue to mostly use the phrase 'social capital' only in a doubly restricted sense, first as referring to the networks which enable individuals to access the human capital and only in a secondary sense the economic capital of others, in the sense of Bourdieu and Coleman; and second solely in regard to how individuals use such networks for their own or their families' and associates' 'private' purposes, and not how they may use such networks for the benefit of their employers in negotiating with other organizations or divisions of organizations, as against Granovetter's presentation of 'embeddedness'. This does not preclude drawing further parallels with wider social phenomena of generalized trust and altruism as envisaged by Putnam (1993a), Etzioni (1993) and Fukuyama (1996) when appropriate.[9]

An example drawn from two pages of Putnam's discussion of the concept of social capital may illustrate why we adopt this approach. Putnam states that in his approach, 'Social capital . . . refers to features of social organisations, such as trust norms, and networks, that can improve the efficiency of society by facilitating coordinated actions' (Putnam 1993a: 167), and he proceeds to cite a passage from Coleman taken from a few pages after the one which we have given.[10] His example concerns farmers baling hay, which involves the use of both skilled labour and equipment. This is an example which does match our definition and which can be seen as a situation in which social capital creates the possibility for a win-win situation: farmers necessarily have excess capacity of labour and skills in order to meet deadlines and emergencies in their own farms; if there is trust then these can be provided to neighbours when not needed free or at cost, whereas commercial provision of emergency services would be prohibitively expensive. On the next page Putnam positively cites as an example of social capital mutual credit societies amongst Javanese peasants. But his depiction of the means by which social pressure is exercised to ensure compliance suggests that this is not an example of social capital, but of the lack of it, in the sense that either banks do not exist, or do not trust peasants, or are not trusted by peasants, so that peasants are forced to have recourse to the methods he describes.[11] The first situation is one which would continue within any healthy farming community, and to which analogies can be imagined within urban contexts, whereas the second is only relevant to a developmental or deprivation context and would cease to be relevant in a different institutional framework, but more importantly it also involves institutions and sanctions which seem to presuppose mistrust rather than trust on a continuous ongoing basis.

Social capital and the circulation of resources

On reading the literature concerning 'social capital' (see Woolcock 1998 for an excellent bibliographic introduction), it becomes apparent that the concept has enormous ramifications and that there seem to be huge problems in separating out the levels on which it is used. As we understand the literature, it seems that it would be legitimate to begin by suggesting that there are at least four mutually influencing and patterning levels. There is no basic 'originary' level, so we will begin with the 'uppermost' and work 'down', although this procedure is arbitrary and in part flows from the fact that the specific area of social capital with which we are concerned is located – by us – on the 'lowest' level. These four levels we will characterize as those of practices, institutions, networks and performance.

The first level would appear to consist of the practices, habits, concepts and expectations that embody and express the level of trust within society. By practices we understand the schemas of behaviour which in fact occur within a society and are classifiable by the members of that society in terms of known types of behaviour. By habits we understand the tendency of particular individuals to react in stereotyped ways in recurrent contexts. By concepts we understand the ways in which these practices and habits are classed in the thought of the society. By expectations we understand the assumption that certain results or patterns of results are likely to follow from any initiated action. Already on this level we encounter the problem that what is social capital from the recipient's point of view may not be seen in this way by the doer or donor. Thus the habit of helping a neighbour in a daily domestic task can arise from feelings of duty or pity without any expectation of reciprocity either direct or 'generational', but for the recipient it is significant whether there are more or less of such persons resident in the neighbourhood.

The second level is that of the institutions which create and preserve levels of trust. These may be spontaneous or formal, horizontal or vertical, consensual or contested, unitary or fragmented. The problem at this level is that through the continuum of reliability and predictability, trust shades into power, in so far as both are preferable to chaos and uncertainty and thus serve to reduce 'transaction costs'.[12] This is the level on which the 'embeddedness' of Karl Polanyi (Polanyi 1944 and see Mingione 1991: 3–32) and of Granovetter (Granovetter 1985, see especially pp. 487–93 [1992: 58–63], 'Embeddedness, Trust and Malfeasance') is most relevant as the necessary context and concomitant of formal organization. Collier suggests that public action can create trust, for instance by facilitating publication of credit ratings, in contexts where otherwise credit-giving agencies will discriminate on the basis of ascriptive characteristics, giving rise to mutual mistrust (Collier 1998: 24–5). The extent to which people will entrust their children, their homes or their possessions to the care of others is a function not only of their estimation of the trustworthiness of the individual but also of the reliability of wider social sanctions against persons who fail in this trust. A loss of confidence in such institutions can therefore initiate a breakdown in reciprocity between individuals even though they have no specific reason to trust each other less.

The third level is that of networks. On one level society can have densities of networks that are measurable and can be correlated with desired welfare outcomes. On another level individuals each have a particular network which constitutes their individual social capital and for which different individual scores can be assigned by adopting a given cut-off level of attenuation, even though most such networks could be pursued to infinitesimal lengths. This seems to us to map onto the use of the term by Bourdieu,[13] although he does not appear to extend measurement of this individual social capital to the following level of the content of services available through the networks. On this level are to be situated the distinctions between weak and strong ties (see Granovetter 1973). This is also the level on which we would probably situate the interstitial version of 'embedding' described by Burt in which specific market relationships are subverted by embedding in a more particular non-market relationship (Burt 1992: 233–6). Your network of social capital exists only in action, so that your knowledge of who you can ask for a favour or for advice, directly or indirectly, is always limited by the extent to which the persons you mix with have shared such knowledge among themselves.

The fourth level is that of the performances, that is, the actual services that the individual does or can acquire through networks of social capital. The security offered by expectations of assistance can be as important for daily life as the assistance actually received. We would also want to situate at this level 'unactualized' social capital, that is, services which individuals could receive from other individuals within their networks, but which do not take place, because of mutual ignorance of the specific needs and capabilities of the network members. This 'informational' deficit may be correlated with, but should not be simply identified with, a deficit in 'social capital' itself, understood as patterns of relationships or levels of trust. This is the level at which human or economic capital is actually set into motion by social capital, even if only in the form of an explicit guarantee.

There are interactions between all of the levels identified, whereby different schools of social and political thought will pick out some as particularly significant and ascribe them particular directions. We take up the question of what services can actually be rendered between dyadic individuals, within structured networks, or in an open community context. Whatever the means, institutions, and expectations of closure, reciprocity with various levels of constraint and sanction, the basis for the existence of social capital, must be weakened by a lessening of the potential basis of services actually provided through the channels of social capital. This may occur not because of any lack of trust but either because there is less capacity to provide such services or because of informational problems in identifying the possibility of provision of such services. It is this problem to which we will later return in the context of Schumpeterian 'creative destruction' and other scenarios of rapid technological and infrastructural change.

We are not in a position to offer any finally worked out theory of social capital. We consider that it is perfectly legitimate to follow up the research programme derived from the work of Putnam (Putnam 1993b: 41–2), which operates on the level of investigating correlations of economic success and social welfare on regional or national levels, with levels of trust measured directly and by various proxies. The causality underlying these correlations is still under dispute, with several factors which have been proposed as causative or formative being regarded by others as jointly produced by some still unidentified factors, such as membership of social organizations and years of education, see Glaeser (2000).

It can be seen that there is ample scope for a project of mapping the mechanisms of social capital onto an extended version of the research programme of transaction costs. Viewed in this light the theory of Putnam is one of a long line of explanations of religion, law, the state and civil society as fumblings towards the creation of the highest possible level of what evolutionary game theorists would call the 'benign conspiracy'. In this perspective the 'free rider' problem is only one of a continuum of problems arising from the moral hazard of incomplete information.

For the questions that concern us here, we prefer however to use models which, first, retain a connection with human capital as being in some sense the underlying content of social capital (as in Coleman 1988: S97–S102 and in an attenuated form in Coleman 1990: 301–6), and, second, which emphasize the social capital of individuals as concretely existing social networks which give access to specific subsets of the human capital and possibly other forms of capital of other members of the network (as in Bourdieu 1986 and recently restated by Foley and Edwards 1999). We see this as according with the requirement of Woolcock, that 'any definition of social capital should focus on its sources rather than its consequences, on what it is rather than what it does' (Woolcock 2000: 9). In this context trust is relativized as only one of the possible mechanisms of social capital formation.

Social capital and closure

The basic structure of social capital seems to consist of the patterns of behaviour, contact and communication that make it possible for individuals to make use of the human capital of other individuals in an informal way, not based purely on economic exchange or on entitlement. The first precondition of this is that other individuals should have skills or knowledge that are useful to others. The second is that there should be a basis for the informal drawing on this resource by others, either on the basis of reciprocity or of membership of a real or imagined community. The third is that there are direct or indirect contacts through which the individuals concerned can identify and communicate with each other.

Unlike human capital, social capital has up to very recently never been the object of conscious investment. It is something that arises of itself between individuals in autonomously evolving contexts and situations. Having identified social capital as something that some communities apparently lack, or in which they are relatively deficient, governments and other agencies have attempted to foster the development of social capital, or to preserve it from attrition.[14] Governments attempt to deploy powerful policy tools through which they can influence education, housing, or community permanence but there is no guarantee that outcomes will be either productive or benign. Whereas Knack did find a positive relationship between generalized trust and economic growth (Knack 2000), he found that there was little positive association between this generalized trust and membership in associations as supposed by Putnam (1993a). In fact in some cases he found the paradoxical result that 'Putnam' associations, those which Putnam supposed to be trust and social-capital forming, had a negative correlation with economic growth, while 'Olson' associations, the kind of sectoral bodies which Olson (1982) associated with restrictive practices and protectionism, had a positive correlation. Knack concludes that we must look more deeply at the unintended consequences of organizations, since a trade union, professional body or trade association, however, 'selfish' their aims may be, will also generate trust and other forms of social cohesion.[15]

One of the preconditions of the working of networks of social capital can be characterized as the ability of individuals to identify and contact other individuals having the skills or knowledge that they lack.[16] One part of this precondition can be met whenever there are groups of individuals in frequent contact who between them embody a heterogeneous mix of skills and knowledge. There is therefore an obvious problem whenever social differentiation leads to the segregation of groups along the lines of skill and knowledge. This would lead to some forms of skill and knowledge only being accessed through the market and through the services of the state and NGOs, while others become completely unavailable. A different form of problem arises when there is a decline in social contacts within groups, so that individuals lack the knowledge of what skills and knowledge others do have.

These classes of problem can be compounded when individuals do not have a sufficiently stable social profile for others. Primarily, this would mean that individuals do not have knowledge of what skills and knowledge others have. Further, there is a lack of that kind of trust which gives rise to reciprocity or to the recognition of community; and finally, that there are inadequate points of contact to generate either of the foregoing. One obvious way in which this has historically given rise to relative deprivation is in the anonymity of large cities. Migratory and fluctuating populations, lacking a prior background of community, only gradually develop the depth and frequency of contacts and trust necessary to give rise to the process of social capital building.[17]

A new danger which would give a further twist to this process can therefore be seen in any acceleration of the rate of technological change and the associated effects of the use of new information and transportation technologies. Individuals are both constrained and explicitly encouraged to adapt to the need to change their way of life and their professional orientation several times during their active lifetime. Individuals must either spend more time commuting or move towards the location of new employment opportunities, in either case disrupting their commitments in their place of origin. Frequent change in the location and line of work combine with the availability of easy and cheap communication and transport, to encourage individuals to maintain contact with persons living at a distance. The maintenance of personal networks over a distance must involve a reduction of the time and effort available for the creation of new networks in their immediate locality. At the same time economic constraints, the effects of public housing policies, and the targeted marketing of new housing developments mean that neighbourhoods become more homogeneous. In terms of social capital the return on investment in local networks is therefore reduced since the mix of skills and knowledge available is low. Since ease of transport and communication reduces the incentive to create new local contacts, those skills and knowledges that are present locally may remain hidden and untapped because of insufficient awareness.

The policy problems associated with social capital flow from what has been said. Although the maintenance of networks of social capital uses real resources, investment in social capital by individuals is not a conscious decision. Making resources available to individuals does not ensure that these will be invested in social capital. There will only be a real increase in the level of social capital where there are policies and frameworks which incentivize each portion of the virtuous circle of fixing identity, making contacts, drawing an advantage from accessing the skills and knowledge of these contacts, and reciprocating (individually or on the community level). Attempts by government and other agencies to substitute for the positive effects of genuine social capital are mostly ineffective and may create new bureaucracies.

Social capital and creative destruction

The development of new technologies leads to the obsolescence not only of artefacts but also of physical and social infrastructures. In 'modern' society there has been a succession of dominant transport and communications technologies and a corresponding succession of waves of decline and obsolescence affecting the infrastructures built up to supply, maintain and service these technologies. This is why the entrepreneurial activity described by Schumpeter in the phrase 'creative destruction' occurs not merely in erratic 'gales', but in identifiable 'waves'. The capital value of infrastructures designed to service one leading technology is written off as a competing technology displaces it. The effects of new technologies do not remain confined to the area or sector within which they were originally developed. They extend to many others, as new uses are found and, particularly as in processes analogous to the sociological concept of 'tipping', demand for products of old technologies falls below a threshold level and decline becomes collapse.

The nature of the leading technologies also has an effect on the bundling of other forms and sectors of production. The dominant forms of power supply, construction, transport and communication displace their rivals with implications for the methods of production, storage and distribution of many other goods. The dominant forms of industrial organization tend to set patterns for the wider labour market. The skills in use in the dominant sectors tend to be seen as generic skills and other skills become the preserve of specialists. Therefore the substitution of one leading technology by another is a process which is accompanied by the creation, destruction and revolutionizing of many other economic sectors.

Throughout history there have been similar waves, associated with the spread of new military and agricultural paradigms that can be seen to be ultimately dependent on the use of new metals and traction animals. Often the change, however, has not followed on immediately from the discovery of the new metal or the domestication of new species but from the invention of some minor technology that suddenly made the basic resource more easily exploitable (in the case of the horse, militarily: the stirrup; in agriculture: the harness which allows horses to be used for ploughing and traction). The advent of modern capitalist production has institutionalized a system of entrepreneurial search for competitive advantage that accelerates the development of new technologies. Although this gives rise to much incremental change, there have been waves of revolutionary change which are associated with steam and canals, coal and railways, oil and automobiles, and electricity and digitized communication.

In the cities of early capitalism, different social classes lived in physical proximity. Although there was intense spatial segregation by street and class or caste consciousness regulating social contact, the skills and knowledge which constitute social capital were accessible to most individuals through intermediaries, if not directly. It is generally conceded that the overall effect of modern transport and communication technologies has been to allow greater degrees of physical segregation of different social strata. Entrepreneurs, members of the liberal professions, state officials, shop and service workers and skilled employees in turn have been liberated from the need to live near to their workplace, their 'constituency' or their market, by the increased ease of travel, storage and communication. This has led to the concentration of such groups in relatively homogeneous suburbs, new towns and urbanized villages.

This has been identified as a key factor in the development of inner city 'sink' areas, which are characterized among other things by the absence of social networks linking the more deprived and disadvantaged with others by the social links of everyday contact. When areas begin to 'tip' into becoming deprived, the relatively more privileged will leave. This has become more than a merely statistical effect. Those who leave are not simply reducing an average, but by choosing 'exit' over 'voice' they subtract a disproportionate amount of social capital from the area (Hirschman 1970: 51). Their skills and knowledge are no longer informally available to the remaining residents, and nor are those of the wider circle to which they could have mediated contact. Their leaving may reduce the amenity of the area and thus induce further leaving, leading to a 'decline' of the area ('tipping', which applies equally when there is class or ethnic replacement or when, as in parts of the Northeast of England, there is no replacement at all – depopulation).

For social capital theory, this process is part of the problem that arises from the fact that social capital is a public good and therefore is subject to all of the problems of underinvestment and opportunism to which public goods in general are subject. In the absence of a strong feeling of community, individuals begin, perhaps unconsciously, to calculate the costs and benefits of contributing to social capital. Uncertainty about the future is in itself a strong factor reducing any likely positive payoff. It therefore produces an unwillingness to 'invest' which further decreases the future payoff.

Social capital and cyberspace

Despite the propagation of differing views by 'cyber-utopian' writers, there seems no reason to suppose that current developments in Information and Communication Technologies will reverse this trend, since any increased investment of social capital by persons liberated from the drudgery of commuting by the development of teleworking will benefit their already socially segregated neighbourhood.[18] The users of cyber-space are currently the relatively privileged. These are the people who are likely to use any improved or cheapened means of communication for keeping in touch with distant family, friends, and colleagues. If they do use it for the purposes of the local PTA, church or clubs this will have the effect of excluding those who are not connected and decreasing the use of other channels of communication.

The less skilled on the other hand are and will be increasingly employed in the service trades. These trades are by nature locational and if the privileged are enabled to work from home, service trades will move to the areas where they live.

'Cyber' home-working could therefore have the effect of abolishing commuting for the privileged while initiating a new wave of commuting of service workers into those villages, suburbs and renewed inner-city areas that are inhabited by home-workers.[19]

There is a growth of a kind of social capital *within* cyberspace, in the form of voluntary mutual assistance through user groups and advice posters. This may have a further negative effect on social capital organized in local spaces, especially if cyber-contacts lead to long-distance visits to initiate real contact. Most of the kinds of social capital which are created within cyberspace should in any case probably be regarded as variants of the embeddedness which exists within particular occupational categories to exchange knowledge about a joint activity. Rather than creating a permanent system of exchange of skills and knowledge, they act primarily as induction mechanisms between individuals who are more or less knowledgeable within a given field of knowledge. The payoff for the givers in this relationship is that new entrants do not tie up excessive amounts of resources (processing time, cable links) while learning how to use the system, or conversely give in to discouragement. Some are of course Coleman's opinion leaders for whom the acquisition and dispensation of knowledge is part of their bid to form the opinions of those they assist (Coleman 1990: 317).

A further threat to the investment of social capital arises from the increasing speed of succession of waves of creative destruction. By reducing the fixity of any social network this acceleration prevents the development of social bonds in number and depth, and prevents the formation of public identities that would be the basis for the formation of such bonds. As argued by Coleman, investment in social capital, whether or not consciously conceived as such, will only take place where a sufficient level of confidence exists, whether this takes the form of trust in others or trust in institutions, which is generated by the existence of closure, patterns of constraints or sanctions which ensure that free riding is kept within tolerable limits, so that contributors will achieve a payoff adequate to motivate them to contribute again (Coleman 1988: S105–S108; 1990: 318–20).

Social capital and social identity

Waves of creative destruction have generally been associated with the appearance of particular leading technologies within the narrow national markets of early capitalism. The super-profits or quasi-rents which accrued to those who developed or entered new technologies at the beginning, combined with the difficulty of financing and organizing the installation of infrastructures such as the canal, railway, tram and automobile networks meant that waves of creative destruction were spaced out to encompass the lives of one or several generations.

The situation in the current global world market is different. Investment is now, in any case, often planned to be written off in ten, five or three years. Many institutional investors are committed to increasing short-term returns rather than to the long-term value of their stocks. The existence of a global capital market means that capital can be much more easily raised for projects that would entail the destruction of the value of existing investments.

The corollary of this is a situation in which for the majority of workers, employment will no longer be a source of a lifelong social identity. During the last 150 years the model of the male skilled and semi-skilled worker pursuing a career in a particular craft or trade has been the paradigm within which the unskilled, the casually employed and the long-term unemployed have been accommodated as marginal discrepancies. Forms of social organization, insurance, education and arguably marriage and the family (and therefore housing) have been built around this central paradigm. The workplace and the organizations centred on it were central to the ethos of the individual. This model may never have extended to the total lifespan of women – in the West – but was nevertheless the paradigm towards which increasing numbers of women were assimilated through this period.

Already in 1947 Robert Merton foresaw identity problems arising from the wholesale reorganization of work and associated loss of transparency of occupational names: 'splintering of work tasks involves *loss of public identity of the job*' ('The machine, the worker and the engineer', *Science* 1947 (105), reprinted Merton 1968: 616–27, esp p. 618.). While neither the profession nor the job-for-life will completely disappear, a new paradigm is now emerging as the leading model, in which constant adaptation to a changing market situation is required. For the older worker and the unskilled this may mean redundancy, casualization and unemployment. For most, however, it will mean a life with a larger number of transitions in which they will be faced with choices that separate them from previous workfellows and throw them together with new ones. This process will give rise to a greater fragmentation of social identity than that produced by a monotonous series of redundancies and re-employments within a single industrial sector, however stressful this may be, especially if mixed with periods of unemployment. Manuel Castells has argued that the flexibilization and fragmentation of the labour market, particularly the increasing dichotomy between a core and peripheral – in his words disposable – labour force, is a more serious source of social disruption than unemployment (Castells 1996: 264–79).

Another way in which technological change has a negative effect on social capital is through the reduction of the usefulness of many practical skills. The art of repair of domestic appliances and installations is being eroded by replaceability on the one hand and regulation requiring professional certification on the other. An increasing number of work-related skills have no direct domestic application. Even the skills of using new ICTs, which are often called on by friends and neighbours, are subject first to rapid devaluation as the technology becomes ubiquitous, and then to rapid obsolescence.

Social capital and the information society

We now need to adapt the measures developed in the various branches of social capital research to apply the concept to the specific problems of the 'information society'. Social capital is perhaps in danger of being confused with social connected-ness. In the model of social integration and social exclusion, the 'excluded' may be seen as losing density of social contact, the most extreme case being the neglect of the elderly in Western societies. While there are certainly correlations here, the exclusion of individuals from active participation in the central social arenas of work, education, politics, leisure and consumption cannot be mapped directly onto social isolation in terms of human contact. This is even more the case with social capital. Those who live in communities where social capital networks do not contain much variety (whether this is because of low variety in the entire neighbourhood or to the existence of restricted networks, possibly based on social segregation by race, class or age) may not be in any way deficient in human contact, but may have continuous and widespread contact with others, who however have no skills or knowledge which the others do not have, and therefore have little to give to each other beyond sociality and co-operation in the most mundane everyday tasks.

However, there can also be areas of low social capital despite the presence of a heterogeneous mix of skills and knowledge. In this case there can be said to be latent social capital which is not finding expression, or an under-investment in social capital. In terms of the paradigms of interest here, there may be various reasons for this: either there is insufficient communication or trust between individuals, or the individuals are not centred in the area but are maintaining networks of contact primarily with individuals elsewhere. In the latter case these networks may be networks of family, friends and colleagues, persons met through direct contact at some previous point in the individual's life, or they may be persons with whom the individual has become associated primarily through new communicational media.

Although we have used much of the conceptualization of social capital developed by Coleman, we do not follow him in extending this term to cover the extent to which parents actively support the learning process of their children. Here it seems to us that at least in 'modern' societies, the level of this involvement is not or is not perceived as being dependent on reciprocation, nor does it generally flow from an obligation which parents feel towards the community (although within underprivileged ethnic groups it could be seen in this light). There is nevertheless a parallel in the problem that he identifies as a possible shortfall between what a parent could and actually does contribute to the child. In his terms, human capital embodied in the parent may be 'irrelevant to the child's educational growth' unless it is 'complemented by social capital embodied in family relations' (Coleman 1988: S110, not taken over into Coleman 1990). In these terms, the problem we are identifying is one where an existing stock of human capital within a geographic area is not (optimally) benefiting the community because of a lack of social capital embodied in social relations.

The additional factor identified as a new threat to the development or maintenance of social capital among those already underprivileged or in danger of social exclusion is an effect of the greater fluidity of social identity. Even allowing for the social homogenization of residential districts, there may be a latent pool of skills and knowledge which does not find expression in the real creation of social capital.

It is difficult to isolate different phases of the cycle of disinvestment, but some processes that feed on each other would be:

- the failure of individuals to identify with an area and thus with the community of that area.
- the absence of a density of contact in everyday life within an area, so that the skills and knowledge which individuals possess do not become known to others.
- the involvements of individuals with others outside the area, whether this is personal contact or contact through new media, leading to lessening of social contact and commitment within the area.
- the disappointment and disruption of expectations of reciprocity due to changing circumstances of others.
- the increasing complication of the indirect mobilization of social capital as the social network of each individual is increasingly spatially spread out.

All of these effects can be seen as symptoms of the disruption of social life by economic change. The argument put forward here is that as the period of return on investment is driven down, these disruptions will increasingly become the normal expected state of affairs. Expectations begin to play a role when investment in social contacts is consciously reduced because of a personal history of disruption caused by redundancy, secondment, plant relocation or career switches. The question which flows from this is whether there are any social policies which can reverse this trend, or whether on the contrary we should accept that social capital will play a reduced role in the future and accept the need to make provision for the supply through the market or the state of even more of the services previously accessed through social networks.

The problem arising from poverty of variety in skills that we are attempting to identify here can perhaps be illuminated by an analogy with the effect of poverty in variety of knowledge on processes of sharing knowledge. Collier (1998), having developed a distinction between the behaviours of 'copying' (adopting the practices of innovators) and 'pooling' (mutual adjustment of the practices of equals) (pp. 8–9), concludes that 'Pooling has more potential to be regressive, because it is intrinsically reciprocal'. Since networks are not open to all, innovators have an incentive to copy among themselves while 'those with little knowledge to share are confined to networking with others with little knowledge and so have less incentive to do so than those with large amounts of knowledge' (Collier 1998: 25).

If social capital is a residual category, and individuals cannot be motivated to make rational decisions to invest in social capital, then the only policies that will be effective in increasing the effective rate of investment in social capital will be those which alter the rate of payoff by increasing the real likelihood of individual or communal reciprocity. Conversely, we know that when patterns of social capital are disrupted, rational decisions lead to counter-productive results as more individuals and families withdraw from networks by physically moving or by reducing reciprocity. Patterns of architecture which pander to these withdrawal decisions make the problem more irreversible. Planners, architects and developers are trapped between designing areas on the assumption of levels of community which do not exist and which therefore invite crime or of designing for levels of withdrawal which are thereby fixed.

Conclusions and indications for future research and for policy

There seems little inclination on the part of policy-makers to attempt to deal with the problems outlined here by attempting to reverse the globalization of markets and thereby reduce the force and frequency of 'waves of creative destruction'. On the contrary, the search for competitive advantage means that national and regional governments wish their areas and locales to be in the forefront of such waves. We can also suppose that the speeding up of waves of technological and infrastructural obsolescence will mean that it will not necessarily be obviously mature or ageing technologies that will be the victims of new developments. We must therefore look for indicators of the ability of social structures to withstand these waves, and at the same time of the ability of individuals to ride them out. In regard to communities this means looking for the factors which encourage 'investment' in social capital. In regard to individuals it means looking for the factors which enable them to make the transitions from one wave to the next. We hope to find some common factors here, so that the health of the community and the success of the nomadic individual may be reconciled.

The most positive recommendation we can provide for policy-makers at community level is to consider the possibility of mobilizing whatever variety of skills and knowledge is available within communities in order to ensure that social networks are able to take full advantage of their potential resource bank. Ways of achieving this end have been discussed by Riel Miller (Miller 1995, developing ideas previously sketched in OECD 1993).

In terms of research we would agree with Willms that the area of social capital research requires 'an integrated set of longitudinal surveys' and that these should examine the 'quality of social relationships' and help to assess 'how social capital affects the processes that are proximal to social outcomes' (Willms 2000: 19–21, esp. p. 19). We would also suggest that social capital research should develop methods of mapping social networks, and particular uses made of social networks, onto the use of various communication technologies and media, and onto spatial and cyberspace locations. Some work in this direction, relating to US data, is found in Bollier 1997 and Katz and Aspden 1998. We intend to work to develop measures of skills and knowledge variety within such networks and locations in order to understand the forms of networking which maximally mobilize the available variety, both for the members of the network and for the wider society.

Notes

1 Largely carried out within the European Commission-funded TSER project COMPETE, Competence Evaluation and Training for Europe, on which see Jones and Hadjivassiliou (1999), building on previous work reported in Cullen and Jones (1997) and DELILAH 1998.

2 Kleinknecht (1987) is a relatively recent defence of the existence of Kondratieff long waves and of the viability of some aspects of Schumpeter's model as a possible explanation of them.

3 See Aghion and Howitt (1997: 231–78), specifically: 'Although each GPT raises output and productivity in the long run, it can also cause cyclical fluctuations while the economy adjusts to it. Examples of GPTs that have affected the entire economic system include the steam engine, the electric dynamo, the laser, and the computer. . . . such GPTs require costly restructuring and adjustment to take place, and there is no reason to expect this process to proceed smoothly over time' (p. 244). '. . . each GPT requires an entirely new set of intermediate goods before it can be implemented. The discovery and development of these intermediate goods is a costly activity, and the economy must wait until some critical mass of intermediate components has been accumulated before it is profitable for firms to switch from the previous GPT' (p. 245).

4 Beck (1992: 140–50) following Sklar for the USA (cited p. 150 n. 4), see also Castells (1996) reporting scenarios published by the US Bureau of Labor Statistics projecting that for the period 1990–2005, US manufacturing output would increase by 2.3% annually while manufacturing employment would fall by 0.2% annually.

5 'The labor market, by way of occupational mobility, place of residence or employment, type of employment, as well as the changes in social location it initiates, reveals itself as the driving force behind the individualization of people's lives. They become relatively independent of inherited or newly formed ties (e.g. family, neighbourhood, friendship, partnership). *There is a hidden contradiction between the mobility demands of the labor market and social bonds*' (Beck 1992: 94).

6 See Becker (1993, especially pp. 85–94), 'The Incentive to Invest' on individual incentives and pp. 23–25 'Human Capital and Economic Development' on the incentive for societies to invest in human capital.

7 Coleman (1990: 304) states clearly: 'The distinction between human capital and social capital can be exhibited by a diagram . . . which represents the relations of three persons (A, B, and C); the human capital resides in the nodes, and the social capital resides in the lines connecting the nodes. Social capital and human capital are often complementary. . . . There must be human capital held by A and social capital in the relation between A and B (in order for B to benefit).' This seems to us to represent the paradigmatic situation in networks of social capital, although in some instances access to economic capital in physical or financial form is also mediated by social capital. In his further investigation of the structures of closure, obligation and trust, Coleman continues to build on this basic cell (Coleman 1990: 304–20).

8 Discussed under the term 'embeddedness' by Granovetter (1985).

9 There is considerable value in the swapping of identical services, looking after children, shopping, giving lifts, waiting for deliveries, etc. This would be valuable even if done on the basis of strict reciprocity of identical services, since the need for such favours arises from the different patterns of demands on the time of individuals concerned. There can be similar reciprocity in joining in activities which can only be carried out by a group; the donors at one time expecting a similar service at another. The reciprocity, or

in Coleman's technical term 'closure', expected may be purely individual-to-individual (with multiple 'accounting systems' whereby a debt of A to B of type X will not necessarily cancel against a debt from B to A of type Y) or within a closer 'community' it may be a more diffuse expectation that one or more group members will make themselves available when necessary. Without undervaluing this kind of social capital, we restrict ourselves to cases of the exchange of unlike services because the exchange of unlike services is more likely to create networks crossing other social divides. The established networks of this kind of exchange are also more liable to disruption by technological change and specifically by the mass obsolescence of the skills of one industrial paradigm when it is replaced by another.

10 'Like other forms of capital, social capital is productive, making possible the achievement of certain ends that would not be attainable in its absence . . . In a farming community, . . . where one farmer got his hay baled by another and where farm tools are extensively borrowed and lent, the social capital allows each farmer to get his work done with less physical capital in the form of tools and equipment' (Putnam 1993a: 167, quoting from Coleman 1990: 302–7).

11 'So strong can be the norm against defection that members on the verge of default are reported to have sold daughters into prostitution or committed suicide' (Putnam 1993a: 168).

12 This is the general thrust of the review of Putnam (1993a) by Levi (1996), see especially pp. 51–2.

13 See Bourdieu (1980 and 1986), the restatement Bourdieu and Wacquant (1992: 119): 'Social capital is the sum of the resources, actual or virtual, that accrue to an individual or a group by virtue of possessing a durable network of more or less institutionalised relationships of mutual acquaintance and recognition', and the investigation of Bourdieu (2000), especially p. 12 and note 2. We cannot here enter into a discussion of the value of Bourdieu's other concepts, cultural capital and symbolic capital.

14 Most prominently in recent years the concept of 'social capital' has been taken up by the World Bank and the OECD. The web sites of these organizations now contain a large amount of literature on social capital theory and the problems of developing or encouraging the development of social capital in a wide range of contexts. The problem for much of the work concerning social capital in the developing world appears to revolve around the question of whether it is possible to develop 'social capital' exclusively from the ground up, in the area of civil society and everyday life. For many societies an absence of social capital may have its ultimate origin in the failure of provision of social capital at the level of the state, law, markets and money, in the form of a predatory state, inadequate availability or even-handedness of legal institutions, missing markets, and money which is either subject to hyper-inflation or which is not in itself an adequate claim to goods.

15 Knack (2000) reports on earlier work published in Knack and Keefer (1997). While this contrast is enlightening, Knack's view perhaps overlooks the specifically efficiency-enhancing activities such as education, training, information pooling and service provision which are part of the selling pitch of 'Olson' organizations, see Olson (1965: 17–35) and Olson (1982: 132–67).

16 On the level of our understanding of individual social capital, following Bourdieu, the 'individual' here should be taken as potentially situated within a network of social capital whereby the provision of knowledge about the knowledge and skills of others is one of the services which members might render one another. The extent to which such information, or fora for the public display of such information, can usefully be mediated by state or NGO bodies (or semi-private institutions such as LETS) is one of the problems which leads into the question of whether all states and markets are not ultimately particular crystallizations of 'social capital'.

17 Migrant groups which retain their original identity are less affected by this problem and may exhibit higher levels of internal social capital under most definitions, while conversely levels of social capital in wider societies may be negatively related to heterogeneity, see Glaeser (2000, section IV), and the conclusion that this is another reason for 'government actions to lessen divides across races or ethnicities' particularly through education policy.

18 For instance, Doheny-Farina (1996: 177–88) advocates mapping virtual social capital onto local social capital, using the web as a local bulletin board, newspaper, and forum, but he does not confront the question of the prior social segregation and self-sorting of populations, taking rural communities as his paradigm. A similar approach is taken by Aurigi and Graham (1998). These authors are not uncritical and raise interesting problems concerning elite and business influence in cyberspace but are basically optimistic about virtual community.

19 Doheny-Farina (1996: 87–96) discusses this phenomenon, reporting that in 1994 there were already 7.6 million tele-workers in the US (p. 91), and millions more who tele-worked from home part-time or evenings.

References

Aghion, P. and Howitt, P. (1997) *Endogenous Growth Theory*, Cambridge, MA: MIT Press.

Aurigi, A. and Graham, S. (1998) 'The "Crisis" in the Urban Public Realm', in Brian D. Loader (ed.) (1998) *Cyberspace Divide*, London: Routledge.

Beck, U. (1992) *Risk Society* (trans. Mark Ritter), London: Sage.

—— (2000) *The Brave New World of Work*, Cambridge: Polity.

Becker, G.S. (1993 [1964]) *Human Capital*, 3rd edn, Chicago: University of Chicago Press.

Bollier, D. (1997) *Social Venture Capital for Universal Electronic Communication*, Washington DC: The Aspen Institute.

Bourdieu, P. (1980) 'Le capital social', *Actes de la recherche en sciences sociales* 31, pp. 2–3.

—— (1986) 'The Forms of Capital', in J.G. Richardson (ed.) *The Handbook of Theory and Research for the Sociology of Education*, New York: Greenwood, pp. 241–58.

—— (2000) *Les structures sociales de l'économie*, Paris: Seuil.

Bourdieu, P. and Wacquant, L. (1992) *An Invitation to Reflexive Sociology*, Cambridge: Polity Press.

Burt, R.S. (1992) *Structural Holes. The Social Structure of Competition*, Cambridge, MA: Harvard University Press.

Castells, M. (1996) *The Rise of the Network Society*, Oxford: Blackwell.

Coleman, J.S. (1988) 'Social Capital in the Creation of Human Capital', *American Journal of Sociology* 94 (Supplement) pp. S95–S120.

—— (1990) *Foundations of Social Theory*, Cambridge, MA: Harvard University Press (see Chapter 12, Social Capital, pp. 300–21).

Collier, P. (1998) *Social Capital and Poverty*, The World Bank Social Capital Initiative Working Paper No. 4.

Cullen, J. and Jones, B. (1997) *State of the Art on Approaches in the United States to Accreditation of Competencies through Automated Cards*, Final report. London: Tavistock Institute Evaluation Development and Review Unit.

DELILAH – *Looking at innovations in education and training. Framework, results, and policy implications of the DELILAH project*. Final Report. Brussels: European Commission 1998. TSER 011.

Doheny-Farina, S. (1996) *The Wired Neighborhood*, New Haven: Yale University Press.

Etzioni, A. (1993) *The Spirit of Community*, New York: The Free Press.

Foley, M.W. and Edwards, B. (1999) 'Is It Time to Disinvest in Social capital?' *Journal of Public Policy* 19, 141–73.

Fukuyama, F. (1996) *Trust*, London: Penguin.

Glaeser, E.L. (2000) *The Formation of Social Capital*, Paper to the International Symposium on The Contribution of Human and Social Capital to Sustained Growth and Well-Being, Quebec City, 19–21 March 2000.

Granovetter, M. (1973) 'The Strength of Weak Ties', *American Journal of Sociology* 78, 1360–80.

—— (1985) 'Economic Action and Social Structure: the Problem of Embeddedness', *American Journal of Sociology* 91, 481–510, reprinted in M. Granovetter and R. Swedberg (eds) 1992, pp. 53–81.

Granovetter, M. and Swedberg, R. (eds) (1992) *The Sociology of Economic Life*, Boulder, Colorado: Westview Press.

Hirschman, A.O. (1970) *Exit, Voice and Loyalty*, Cambridge, MA: Harvard University Press.

Jones, B. and Hadjivassiliou, K. (1999) 'New methods of skills definition and accreditation: personal skills medium in the USA and in Europe', CEDEFOP Experts AGORA Thessalonika March 1999 (Chapter in CEDEFOP publication, *Identification, assessment and recognition of non-formal learning* – forthcoming).

Katz, J. E. and Aspden, P. (1998) *Cyberspace and Social Community Development, Internet Use and its Community Integration Correlates*, http//www.iaginteractive.com/emfa/cybsocdev.htm, 03/05/98.

Kleinknecht, A. (1987) *Innovation Patterns in Crisis and Prosperity. Schumpeter's Long Cycle Reconsidered*, London: Macmillan.

Knack, S. (2000) *Trust, Associational Life and Economic Performance*. Paper to the International Symposium on The Contribution of Human and Social Capital to Sustained Growth and Well-Being, Quebec City 19–21 March 2000.

Knack, S. and Keefer, P. (1997) 'Does Social Capital Have an Economic Payoff? A Cross-Country Investigation', *Quarterly Journal of Economics* 112, 1251–88.

Levi, M. (1996) 'Social and Unsocial Capital: A Review Essay of Robert Putnam's Making Democracy Work', *Politics and Society* 24, 45–55.

Merton, R. K. (1968 [1949]). *Social Theory and Social Structure*, 3rd edn, New York: Free Press.

Miller, R. (1995) *Territorial Development and Human Capital in the Knowledge Economy: Towards a Policy Framework*, Paris: OECD.

Mingione, E. (1991) *Fragmented Societies* (trans. Paul Goodrick), Oxford: Basil Blackwell.

OECD (1993) *Territorial Development and Structural Change*, Paris: OECD.

Olson, M. (1965) *The Logic of Collective Action*, Cambridge, MA: Harvard University Press.

—— (1982) *The Rise and Decline of Nations*, New Haven: Yale University Press.

Polanyi, K. (1944) *The Great Transformation*, Boston: Beacon Press.

Putnam, R. D. (1993a) *Making Democracy Work*, Princeton: Princeton University Press.

—— (1993b) 'The Prosperous Community. Social Capital and Public Life', *The American Prospect*, Spring, 35–42.

Ritzen, J. (2000) *Social Cohesion, Public Policy, and Economic Growth: Implications for the OECD Countries*. Keynote address prepared for International Symposium on The Contribution of Human and Social Capital to Sustained Growth and Well-Being, Quebec City 19–21 March 2000.

Schumpeter, J. (1939). *Business Cycles* (2 volumes). New York: McGraw-Hill. Abridged edition (1964) by Rendig Fels, New York: McGraw-Hill. Reprint of the Abridgement (1989) Philadelphia: Porcupine Press. See the chapters 'How the Economic System Generates Evolution' and 'The Contours of Economic Evolution'.

—— (1961 [1934, 1911]) *Theory of Economic Development* (trans. by Redvers Opie from the 4th German edn). New York: Oxford University Press.

—— (1976 [1942]) *Capitalism, Socialism and Democracy*, London: George Allen & Unwin.

Willms, J. D. (2000) *Three Hypotheses about Community Effects Relevant to the Contribution of Human and Social Capital to Sustaining Economic Growth and Well-Being*. Paper to the International Symposium on The Contribution of Human and Social Capital to Sustained Growth and Well-Being, Quebec City 19–21 March 2000.

Woolcock, M. (1998) 'Social capital and economic development: Toward a theoretical synthesis and policy framework', *Theory and Society* 27: 151–208

—— (2000) *The Place of Social Capital in Understanding Social and Economic Outcomes*. Paper to the International Symposium on The Contribution of Human and Social Capital to Sustained Growth and Well-Being, Quebec City 19–21 March 2000.

Index